Clinico-Pathological
Atlas of Congenital
Fundus Disorders

Juan Orellana • Alan H. Friedman

Clinico-Pathological Atlas of Congenital Fundus Disorders

• With 236 Illustrations •
196 in Color

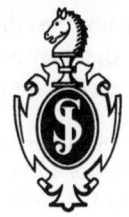

Springer Science+Business Media, LLC

Juan Orellana, M.D., F.A.C.S.
Associate Clinical Professor of Ophthalmology
Mount Sinai School of Medicine
New York, NY 10029, USA

Alan H. Friedman, M.D.
Clinical Professor of Ophthalmology
Mount Sinai School of Medicine
New York, NY 10029, USA

Library of Congress Cataloging-in-Publication Data
Orellana, Juan.
    Clinico-pathological atlas of congenital fundus disorders / Juan
Orellana, Alan H. Friedman.
        p.   cm.
    Includes bibliographical references and index.
    ISBN 978-1-4613-9322-1   ISBN 978-1-4613-9320-7 (eBook)
    DOI 10.1007/978-1-4613-9320-7
    1. Fundus oculi--Diseases--Atlases. 2. Abnormalities, Human-
-Atlases.   I. Friedman, Alan H., 1937-   . II. Title.
    [DNLM: 1. Eye Abnormalities--pathology--atlases. 2. Retinal
Diseases--congenital--atlas.   3. Retinal Diseases--pathology-
-atlases.   WW 17 O66c]
RE545.O74   1993
617.7'4--dc20
DNLM/DLC
for Library of Congress   92-49529

Printed on acid-free paper.

Production managed by Christin R. Ciresi; manufacturing coordinated by Rhea Talbert.
Photocomposed pages prepared from the author's MacWrite II files using QuarkXPress.
Printed and bound by Walsworth Publishing Co., Marceline MO, USA

9 8 7 6 5 4 3 2 1

For my wife, Jeanne,
my children Adam, Nikelle, Jennifer, and Jason,
and my parents, Juan and Rosaura

Preface

Over the many years of practice, countless referrals have been made by ophthalmologists curious enough to ask the question, "What is this?" Ophthalmology being such a visual discipline, we often refer to texts with many illustrations in an attempt to match the lesion to the picture. Once we have found the appropriate match, we can discuss the diagnosis and the ultimate visual prognosis and therapy with the patient.

A great sigh of relief often accompanies the explanation that the lesion is benign, not a malignancy. For some patients the lesions are amenable to therapy, whereas for others a systemic syndrome has been diagnosed that includes ocular manifestations. Appropriate referral can then be made to ensure that the patient will enjoy good health despite having several systems involved.

The purpose of this book is to provide the reader with a concise but extensively illustrated text that points out the salient clinical features of congenital anomalies of the vitreous, retina, and choroid and then correlates these features with the associated pathology. The book has been divided into sections dealing with various aspects of vitreoretinal disorders including genetic, vascular, infectious, and neoplastic entities. The subject of pathology (as much as possible) has been included because to truly understand the implications of a disease, its therapy, and its prognosis, its pathology must be understood. Therapy and visual prognosis have been included to complete the discussions. We have included the angiographic and ultrasonographic findings wherever possible. These ancillary tests often help in the differential diagnosis of fundus disorders. Selected references have been included to enable the reader to research the topic in more depth. Many excellent references have been omitted for lack of space, although their contributions have been included in the text.

As with any other discipline, to decipher a problem one must be versed in the steps and methods needed to solve the puzzle. In this case, it means that the reader should be familiar with anatomy and embryology, ocular genetics, basics of pathology and methods of examination used in adults and children. This information forms the foundation on which the rest of the book is based.

Contents

Section 10. Tumors

Section 11. Miscellaneous Disorders

Section 1

Elementary Principles

Chapter 1

Anatomy and Embryology

The neural ectoderm expands as the embryo grows and ultimately forms two folds with a midline groove. The folds come together, forming a tube that is commonly called the neural tube. Bilateral thickenings at the cephalic end of this tube are the beginnings of the eye. With further development the thickenings become optic pits and finally optic vesicles. The optic vesicle now harbors the cells needed to form an eye. The central portion gives rise to the sensory retina and the lateral portions to the iris epithelium and ciliary body. The outermost part of the vesicle becomes the pigment epithelium. Overlying the optic vesicle is the surface ectoderm, which eventually gives rise to the lens.

By day 25 the neural tube is closed, and an optic vesicle is formed. The lumen of the vesicle communicates with the third ventricle. The sides of this lumen at the vesicle ultimately become the optic stalk. The combination of lens placode and sensory retina have invaginated to produce the lens and optic cup, with the vitreous cavity separating these two structures. It is here that we see formation of the choroidal fissure, which ends anteriorly as the pupil and posteriorly with transit of the central retinal artery into the eye. (Fig. 1-1)

Vitreous

The vitreous body is formed during three phases. Initially, the primary vitreous begins to form at about 21 days' gestation and continues to the ninth week. It appears to be connected to the Müller cell footplates and by the ninth week has become responsible for initial vasoformation. Part of the tunica vasculosa lentis anteriorly and the hyaloid system along with the central retinal artery are derived from the mesodermal cells of the primary vitreous. The collagen fibrils and hyalocytes are seen as the secondary vitreous rises from the sensory retina or perhaps from the primary vitreous itself. The secondary vitreous grows around the primary vitreous, forcing the primary vitreous into the center to form the walls of Cloquet's canal. The secondary vitreous also extends from the equatorial lens to the iris and forms the bed from which the tertiary vitreous travels after originating from the retinal cells. The primary and secondary vitreous, which remain in contact with the lens, become the hyaloideocapsular ligament. This ligament defines the retrolental space of Berger in which cells are seen in conditions such as retinitis pigmentosa. The hyaloideocapsular ligament is strong in children and young adults but weakens with age. This phenomenon was witnessed in the days of intracapsular cataract surgery. Enzyme (α-chymotrypsin) was used to help weaken the ligaments and zonules, thereby enabling cataract surgery without loss of vitreous.

Anatomy

Anatomically, the vitreous has strong attachments to the retina in several areas. The attachments are at the optic nerve, blood vessels, macula, the back of the lens, and the peripheral retina-ora serrata. Occupying more than two thirds of the globe's volume, it is about 4 ml in volume with a weight of 4 g. It is most firmly anchored straddling the ora serrata, varying in width from 2 to 5 mm or more. This portion forms the vitreous base. The vitreous here is denser than in the center or posteriorly. The vitreous attaches to the internal limiting membrane of the posterior pole by fine collagen fibrils. Intermingled in the vitreous are the hyalocytes. By the seventh month of gestation, blood flow in the hyaloid artery ceases.

Histology

The solid vitreous contains collagen fibrils, peripheral cells (hyalocytes), and proteins. The liquid portion of the vitreous is composed mostly of water but also has inorganic salts, ascorbic acid, hyaluronic acid, proteins and sugar. The collagen fibrils are concentrated in the vitreous cortex and arranged in a random pattern. They appear to arrange themselves at right angles to the vitreous base. The central vitreous does not have nearly the number of fibrils as does the cortex.

Hyalocytes have lobulated nuclei with Golgi complexes and secretory granules in the cytoplasm. Adult vitreous has more hyalocytes than does fetal vitreous. These cells may play a role in the manufacturing of hyaluronic acid, which is found concentrated around collagen fibrils.

Retina

The outer layer of the optic cup in the 1-month-old embryo becomes the retinal pigment epithelium (RPE). Melanin production begins early and by the second month of gestation (proceeding from the posterior pole anteriorly) a basement membrane is secreted by these cells. The outer layer of this membrane (Bruch's) is secreted by the choriocapillaris. The developing pigment epithelium apparently is important, as it stimulates development of the neurosensory retina, choroid, and sclera.

We have seen that the optic cup has neuroectodermal cells. There are two zones here: the primitive and the marginal. Neural and glial cells develop from the center of the cup and progress toward the rim. By the end of the second month there are two nuclear layers with the Müller cells growing as well. The external limiting membrane is present by the second month. Further differentiation of these nuclear layers gives rise to ganglion (the first cells to differentiate and whose axons initiate development of the optic nerve), amacrine, bipolar cells, and photoreceptors. The cones can be recognized by the fourth month, and the rods are seen by the seventh month. The macula is not present until the fifth month and the final topographical appearance of the macula is not seen until after birth.

Anatomy

Anatomically, the retina is thinnest at the fovea; it is thicker in the perifoveal and peripapillary regions. It thins out as it approaches the ora serrata. It is separated from the pigmented retina by a potential space, the intraretinal space. Anteriorly, the sensory retina merges with the nonpigmented ciliary epithelium of the pars plana; and posteriorly, it terminates at the optic nerve. Both points have strong pigment epithelium-sensory retina attachments.

In the posterior pole, the fovea can be found 4 mm temporal and 0.8 mm inferior to the center of the optic nerve. The retina is thin here, as the ganglion cell layer, inner plexiform layer, and nerve fiber layer are absent. The inner nuclear layer is missing in the center of the fovea but becomes evident at the edge of the fovea; it has two nuclei per cell. The foveal avascular zone (FAZ) is 0.4 mm in diameter and is fed by the choriocapillaris found underneath.

In the periphery, the retina is also thin. It ends at the ora serrata, the scalloped structure seen in the periphery that is 2.5 mm wide temporally and about 0.75 mm wide nasally. The retinal vascular system is provided by the hyaloid artery, a branch of the ophthalmic artery. Budding from the hyaloid artery, which forms at the same time as the primary vitreous, are the retinal vessels, seen by the fourth month of gestation. Vascular growth continues toward the ora serrata in the nerve fiber layer reaching the ora at 8 months nasally and 9 months temporally.

Histology

The retinal pigment epithelium is found lying on Bruch's membrane. It is a monolayer of cells with a base applied to the choriocapillaris and an apex pointing toward the photoreceptors (Figs. 1-2 and 1-3). The apical portion of the RPE is composed of villous processes that enfold the outer portion of the photoreceptor. The cytoplasm of the pigment epithelium is composed of a variety of structures including phagosomes which contain portions of phagocytosed photoreceptor discs, melanin granules, lipofuscin, Golgi complex, and a nucleus. The base of the cells has numerous enfoldings.

Overlying the pigment epithelium is the neurosensory retina. It is composed of the photoreceptors, external limiting membrane, outer nuclear layer, outer plexiform layer, inner nuclear layer, inner plexiform layer, ganglion cell layer, nerve fiber layer, and the internal limiting membrane (Fig. 1-4).

Optic Nerve

By the second month of gestation, the axons of the ganglion cells have entered the optic stalk and are traveling toward the brain. The stalk itself has neural crest cells and neuroectodermal cells. The axons travel through this stalk, and gradually the center region gives rise to the hyaloid artery, surrounded by the ganglion cell axons. Some of the stalk's central cells differentiate into glial cells, which form septa between groups of axonal bundles.

Anatomy

Although we call the optic nerve a nerve, it is really a fiber tract running from the eye to the brain. Its fibers are derived from the ganglion cell layer of the retina terminating in the lateral geniculate body. It is about 5 mm in width and covered by meninges. Within the cranial cavity, it is covered only by pia; however in the optic canal the dura (divided into the periorbita and dural covering of the nerve) and arachnoid are added. There are spaces between these layers that allow communication with the cranial cavity. The nerve loses most of its myelin sheath as it passes into the eye at which point there is also a loss of connective tissue. It narrows to a diameter of 1.5 mm inside the eye (from 3.0 mm at its connection to the sclera). The central retinal artery and vein enter the optic nerve 10-12 mm posterior to the sclera. The nerve is 20-30 mm in length from globe to optic canal.

The lamina cribrosa is a dense collection of connective tissue that connect the sclera across the scleral canal. Through it travel the fascicles of the optic nerve. Numerous astrocytes can be seen in the intraocular portion of the nerve.

Histology

The optic nerve has three main components: (1) myelinated nerve fibers; (2) interstitial cells, such as astrocytes, oligodendrocytes, and microglia; and (3) fibrovascular septa of the pia mater. With hematoxylin and eosin (H & E) staining, the optic nerve appears pale and somewhat eosinophilic, with few other cells seen (Fig. 1-5). The optic nerve fibers are actually axons of the retinal ganglion cells. With disease, the axons are lost along with their myelin sheaths.

The astrocytes furnish nutritional support to the nerve fibers. They have a branching pattern that resembles a star. The oligodendrocytes are analogous to the schwann cells of the peripheral nerves. Microglia are the macrophages of the central nervous system.

Choroid

The retinal pigment epithelium is necessary to induce the growth and development of the choroid, which is composed principally of cells derived from the neural crest. After the appearance of the pigment epithelium, nearby mesoderm begins to form the endothelium of the choriocapillaris.

The larger vessels can coalesce into bundles that regroup and form the vortex veins. As veins join, new capillaries are formed to replace them. By the fifth month, the short and long ciliary nerves have entered the choroid, Bruch's membrane is present, and the vortex veins can be seen. From the fifth month on, pigmentation by melanocytes derived from the neural crest proceeds anteriorly.

Anatomy

The choroid is a pigmented vascular uveal tissue that extends from the ora serrata (from the ciliary body, also uveal tissue) to the optic nerve. The choroid is thicker at the posterior pole than at the ora serrata. There is a potential space between the choroid and the sclera called the suprachoroidal space. The choroid is a highly vascular organ with a large volume of blood flowing through its vessels. It nourishes the pigment epithelium and outer retinal structures. The long posterior ciliary arteries enter the globe lateral to the optic nerve and course anteriorly in the suprachoroidal space, where they branch at the ora to supply part of the choriocapillaris. The short ciliary arteries also travel for a short distance in the suprachoroidal space and then branch to supply other parts of the choriocapillaris. Venous drainage is accomplished via the vortex veins. Located closer to the vertical in each quadrant, they usually number one per quadrant, although it is not uncommon to see two in a quadrant. The posterior ciliary nerves provide much of the nervous innervation to the choroid. The choroid is rich in sympathetic and parasympathetic neurons.

Histology

The choroid is separated from the sclera by the suprachoroidal space. The choroid has a stromal and a vascular layer. The stromal layer is composed of pigmented cells (choroidal melanocytes) and nonpigmented cells (fibroblasts). Along with these two types of cell are collagen fibrils and a mucinous ground substance. The vessels of the choroid are composed of a network of large vessels that drain into a capillary bed situated underneath the basement membrane (Figs. 1-6 and 1-7). This capillary bed, called the choriocapillaris, is important because it nourishes the overlying retinal pigment cells. The choriocapillaris and the RPE share a basement membrane—Bruch's membrane.

Selected Reading

Apple DJ, Rabb MF (1991). Ocular Pathology. Clinical Applications and Self-Assessment. 4th Ed. St. Louis: Mosby

Snell RS, Lemp MA (1989). Clinical Anatomy of the Eye. Cambridge: Blackwell

Spencer WH, Font RL, Green WR, et al (1985). Ophthalmic Pathology. An Atlas and a Textbook. 3rd Ed. Philadelphia: Saunders

Yanoff M, Fine BS (1989). Ocular Pathology. A Text and Atlas. 3rd Ed. Philadelphia: Lippincott

Figures

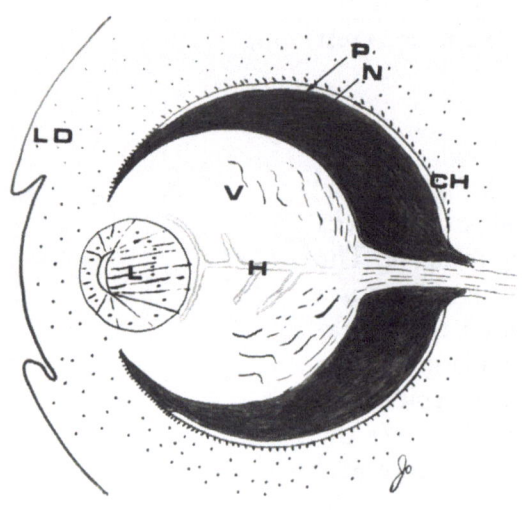

FIGURE 1-1.
Anteroposterior representation of an early (15-17 weeks) fetal eye. Beginning anteriorly are the lids (LD); the lens (L) with its nucleated cells; the hyaloid artery (H) within the vitreous cavity (V); the inner vascular layers (IV); and the pigment (P) and nervous (N) layers of the retina. An early choroid (CH) is developing.

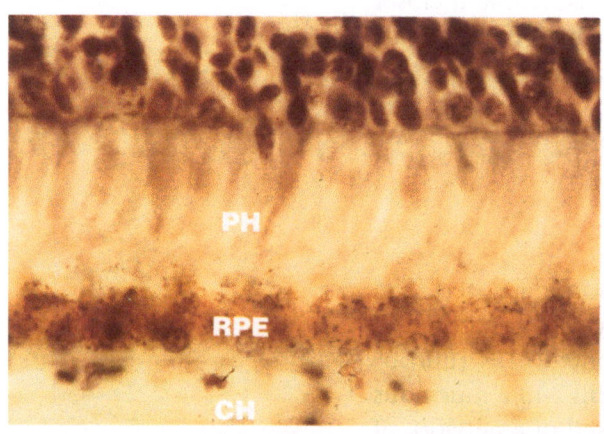

FIGURE 1-2.
Complex consisting of the choriocapillaris (CH), retinal pigment epithelium (RPE), and photoreceptors (PH). (H & E)

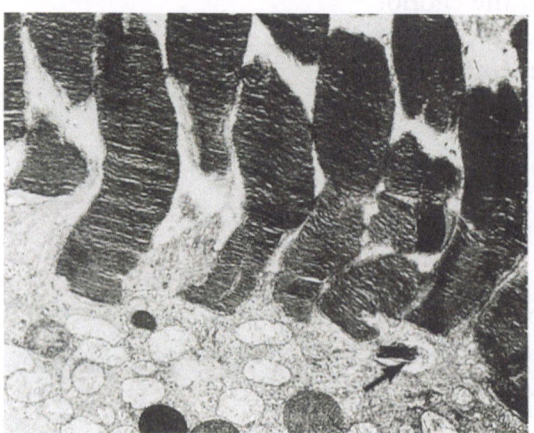

FIGURE 1-3.
Pigment epithelial cells enveloping the photoreceptor discs. Note, at lower right, the phagocystosis of the discs. (arrow) (Electron Micrograph)

FIGURE 1-4.

Layers of the normal adult retina: pigment epithelium (PE); rods and cones (RC); external limiting membrane (ELM); outer nuclear layer (ONL); outer plexiform layer (OPL); inner nuclear layer (INL); inner plexiform layer (IPL); ganglion cell layer (G); nerve fiber layer (NFL); and the internal limiting membrane (ILM). (H & E)

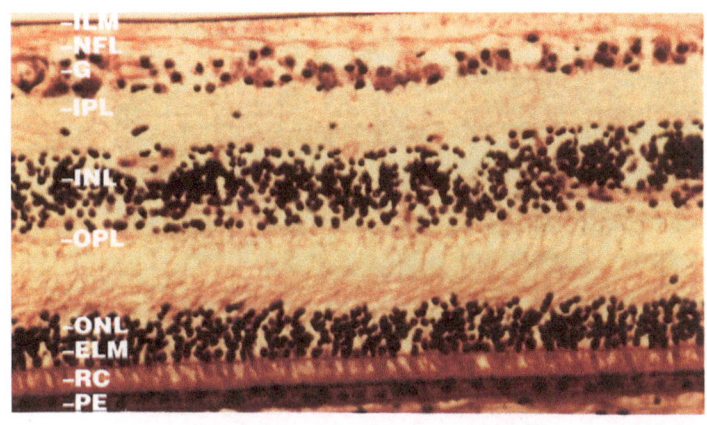

FIGURE 1-5.

Normal optic nerve. The central vessels can be seen in cross section at the top left of the photomicrograph. The cup is normal, and the optic nerve axons can be seen. (H & E)

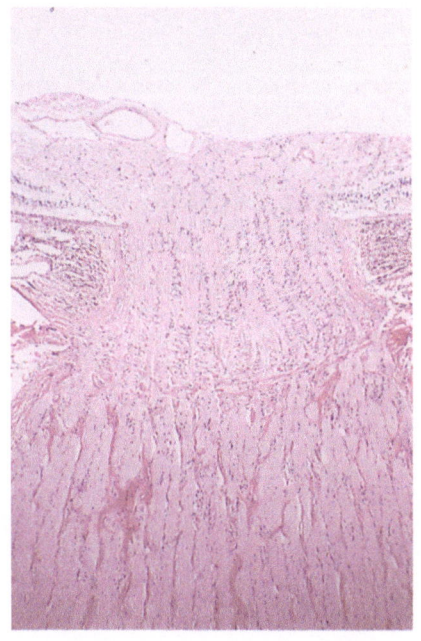

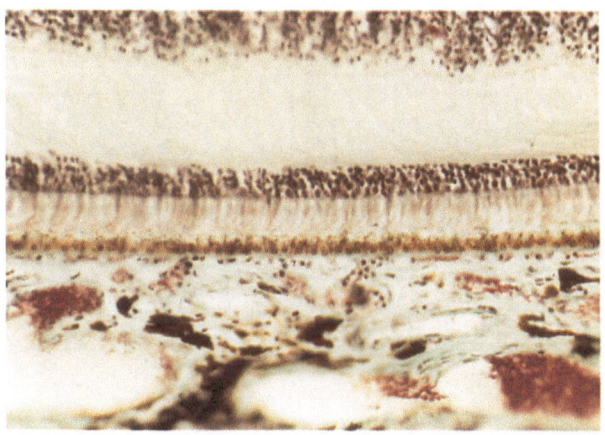

FIGURE 1-6.

Large, medium, and small choroidal vessels, Bruch's membrane, pigment epithelium and outer retina. (Trichrome stain)

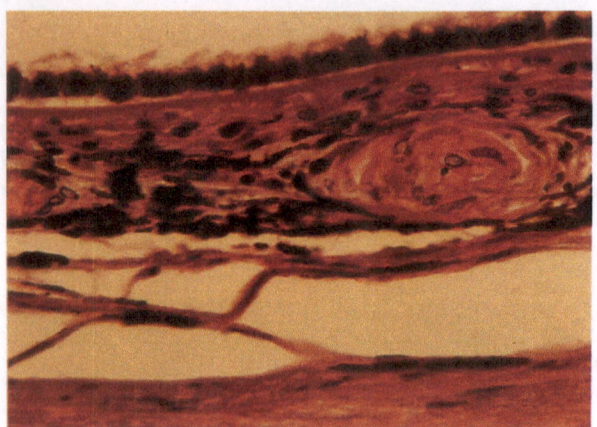

FIGURE 1-7.
Large vessels are seen in the choroid. The pigment epithelium can also be seen at the top of the section. (H & E)

Chapter 2

Basics of Pathology

To appreciate the success achieved at surgery or the resumption of 20/20 vision in the patient, you must have a working knowledge of pathology. The ability to fix presumes that you have an idea of how it works and what has happened to "break" it. Most residents do not appreciate the pathology laboratory until they have left their residency and usually try to take a comprehensive review course at some point in their career.

Essentially, in the pathology laboratory the whole eye is sectioned into three parts: a central, pupillooptic nerve section and two calottes. The external landmarks having been established, the pathologist determines whether the specimen is the right or left eye and whether it is horizontal or vertical. It may be stated, however, the pathologist makes his own determination. The eye may be sectioned horizontally or vertically depending on the preferences or the expected pathology in that particular case. On occasion, transillumination helps determine where, for example, a melanoma is hidden. From here the fixed specimen is prepared for histological study.

Tissues take up stains, which allow details to be readily discerned. The basic working stain is hematoxylin and eosin (H & E) (Fig. 2-1); hematoxylin stains nucleic acids blue, and eosin stains most cytoplasmic organelles pink. After reviewing a specimen slide stained with H & E, the pathologist may want to look at the same slide using a different stain that brings out other characteristics of that tissue sample. For example, periodic acid-Schiff (PAS, Fig. 2-2) stains glycoproteins red; trichrome stains collagen blue (Fig. 2-3); alcian blue tints mucopolysaccharides blue (e.g., those found in vitreous) (Fig. 2-4); myelin stains bluish with Luxol fast blue stain (Fig. 2-5); oil red O stains lipids red (Fig. 2-6); silver stains result in black marking of those tissues that contain melanin or reticular fibers (Fig. 2-7); and the Von Kossa stain causes calcium to appear red (Fig. 2-8). With these few stains, we should be able to understand most pathology of the vitreous, retina, optic nerve, and choroid.

Cellular Components

The cell is organized into nuclear and cytoplasmic portions. The contents are enclosed by a semipermeable membrane called the cell plasma membrane. Within the apparently clear cytoplasm lies colloid rich in organelles. Muscle cells have myofibrils, and epithelial cells have tonofilaments. Mitochondria, which manufacture energy for the cell, are dispersed throughout the cytoplasm. Endoplasmic reticulum, Golgi complex, centrioles, and lysosomes are also found in the cytoplasm. The nucleus harbors the nucleolus and chromatin. In health, a steady state develops between cells that, when upset, produces a disease state.

Cellular Types and Reactions

Cells that react to injury, noxious materials, or bacteria are called polymorphonuclear leukocytes (Fig. 2-9). They are the most numerous of the circulating leukocytes. Within their cytoplasm are numerous lysozymes containing important enzymes. The absence of some enzymes has been linked to congenital diseases such as metachromatic leukodystrophy (absence of arylsulfatase A) or Gaucher's disease (β-glucosidase).

Eosinophils are found in increased numbers when parasites or allergic reactions are present (Fig. 2-10). Basophils mediate the release of heparin and histamine in acute inflammatory reactions. Acutely, the basophils or mast cells cause the passage of cells and fluid from the circulation. This substance is called exudate—serous if the exudate is proteinaceous and purulent if there are many polymorphonuclear neutrophils (PMNs) and necrotic cell debris. The PMNs may summon the macrophages by virtue of a phenomenon called chemotaxis (Fig. 2-11). The macrophages can then transform into epithelioid cells or inflammatory giant cells.

Chronic nongranulomatous inflammation is composed of plasma cells (Fig. 2-12) and lymphocytes (Fig. 2-13), whereas chronic granulomatous inflammation is composed of plasma cells, lymphocytes, and especially epithelioid cells and inflammatory giant cells. Granulomatous inflammation can be one of three types: diffuse, discrete, or zonal. Diffuse reactions may be seen with cytomegalic inclusion disease and toxoplasmosis; and zonal reactions are seen with parasitic infestations. Both types of inflammatory reaction contain lymphocytes. Inflammatory giant cells, which result from fusion of several macrophages, may be found with both diffuse and zonal inflammations.

Reaction Definitions

The terms hypertrophy and hyperplasia are often used incorrectly and are confused with one another. *Hypertrophy* refers to a situation where each element is growing in size, for example, hypertrophy of the corneal nerves in neurofibromatosis (Ch. 44). *Hyperplasia* is different; it indicates a multiplication of elements; for example, hyperplasia of the retinal pigment epithelium after trauma. *Hypoplasia* indicates that the tissue did not fully undergo its scheduled development, for example optic nerve hypoplasia (Ch. 27). *Atrophy* is the decrease in size of the element usually associated with a decrease in function, for example optic atrophy in patients with retinitis pigmentosa (Ch. 37). *Dysplasia* is an abnormal growth of the element as it was developing; coloboma of the retina is an example (Ch. 25). *Neoplasia* is hyperplasia out of control. Hyperplasia attains a growth plateau, where an equilibrium has been attained. With neoplasia, this plateau does not exist, and growth continues. Neoplasia can be benign or malignant. Malignant neoplasia displays the attributes of invasion and metastasis.

There are many types of *necrosis*, but our review of infectious diseases presents us mostly with examples of suppurative necrosis. This type of necrosis is seen with the breakdown of tissue by proteolytic enzymes. Related to it is *putrefaction*, which refers to the change in tissue brought by destructive bacterial enzymes.

Pigmentation is an important element we encounter when dealing with hemorrhage, drusen, or nevi. We need to determine what is melanin, hemosiderin, or lipofuscin. The retinal pigment epithelium (RPE), ciliary body, and iris have large black granules of melanin. Lipofuscin is a pigment seen in both RPE cells and older cells; and it can be seen overlying a choroidal nevus. The oxidation of hemoglobin to hemosiderin after an intraocular bleed can produce hemosiderosis bulbi. The orange brown pigment of hemosiderin is engulfed by the macrophages.

With these explanations of the cell types, reactions, and definitions, the illustrations in the book should be clear to the reader. An understanding of what is wrong at the structural level should help us understand what therapy, if any, can help the patient.

Selected Reading

Apple DJ, Rabb MF (1991). Ocular Pathology. Clinical Application and Self-Assessment. 4th Ed. St Louis: Mosby

Margo CE, Grossniklaus HE (1991). Ocular Histopathology. A Guide to Differential Diagnosis. Philadelphia: Saunders

Spencer WH, Font RL, Green WR, FA, et al (1985). Ophthalmic Pathology. An Atlas and Textbook. 3rd Ed. Philadelphia: Saunders

Stefani FH, Hasenfratz G (1987). Macroscopic Ocular Pathology. An Atlas Including Correlations with Standardized Echography. Berlin: Springer-Verlag

Figures

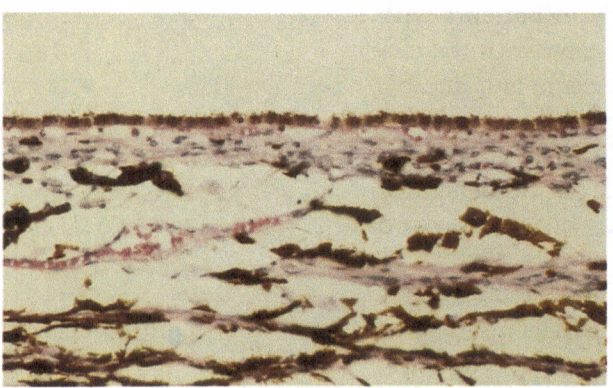

FIGURE 2-1.
Pigment epithelium, choroid, and sclera. in a full thickness eye-wall section. (H & E)

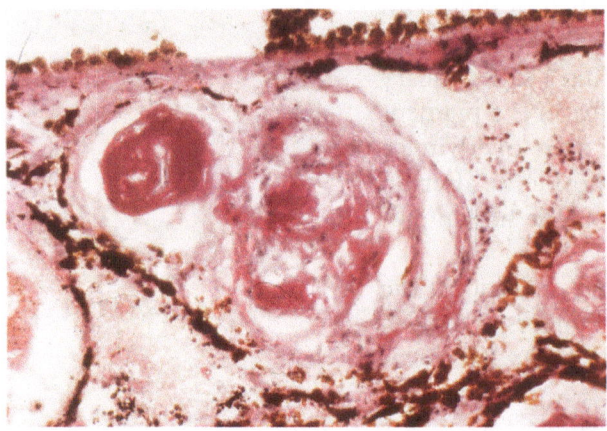

FIGURE 2-2.
Section obtained from a patient who had lupus erythematosus. There is a deposition of fibrinoid material within the choroidal vessels. (PAS)

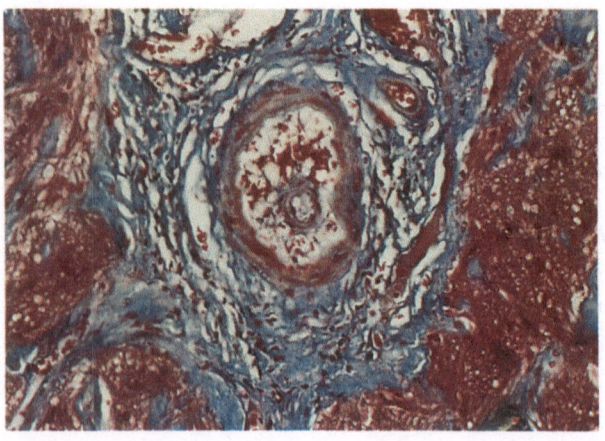

FIGURE 2-3.
Atherosclerosis of the central retinal artery. Note the hemorrhage in the vessel wall. (Trichrome stain)

FIGURE 2-4.
Section of the vitreous demonstrating asteroid hyalosis. Note the aggregates of vitreous deposits stained positively for mucopolysaccharides. (Alcian blue) (arrow)

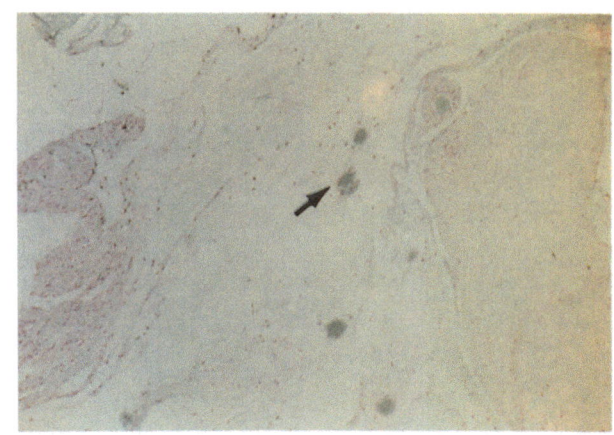

FIGURE 2-5.
Note the myelin in the optic nerve and myelin extruded into the subretinal space in this eye at autopsy. (Luxol fast blue) (arrows)

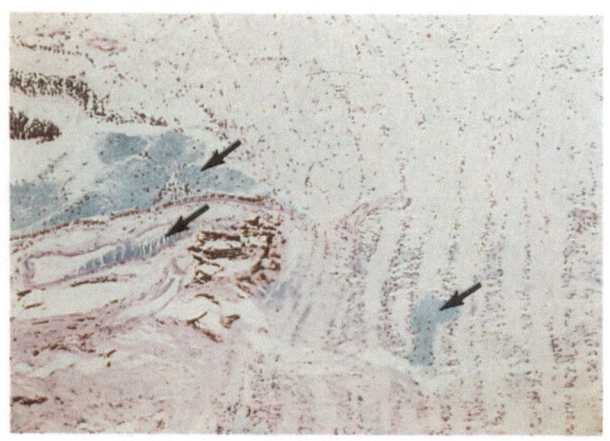

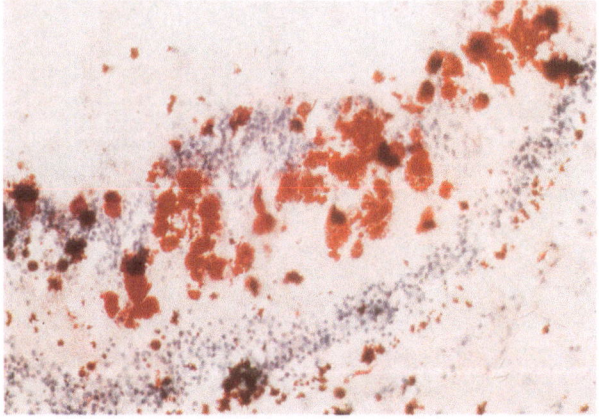

FIGURE 2-6.
Note the lipid in the outer plexiform layer of this retina. (Oil red O; frozen section)

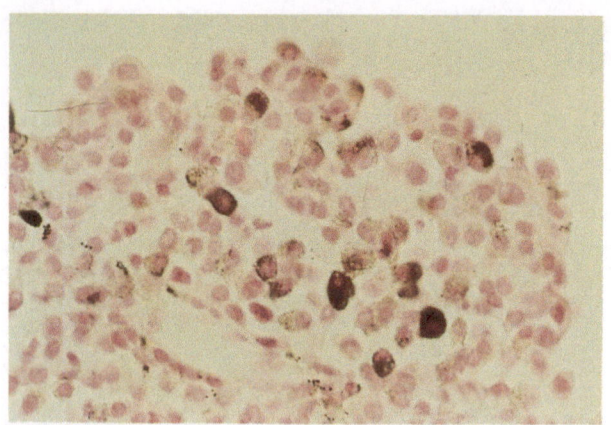

A

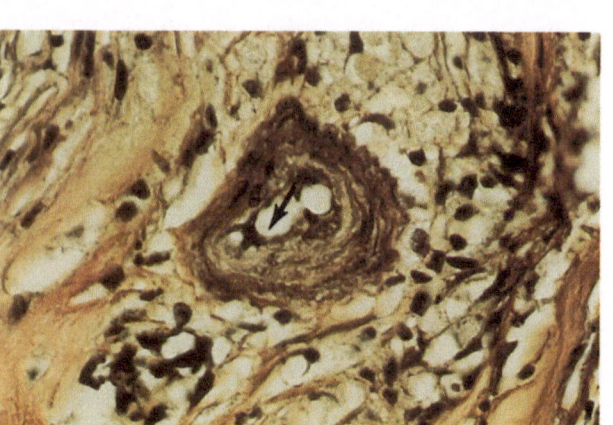

B

FIGURE 2-7.
(A) Melanin granules are inside the macrophages. (B) Note the elastic fibers (arrow) of the central retinal artery. (Silver stain)

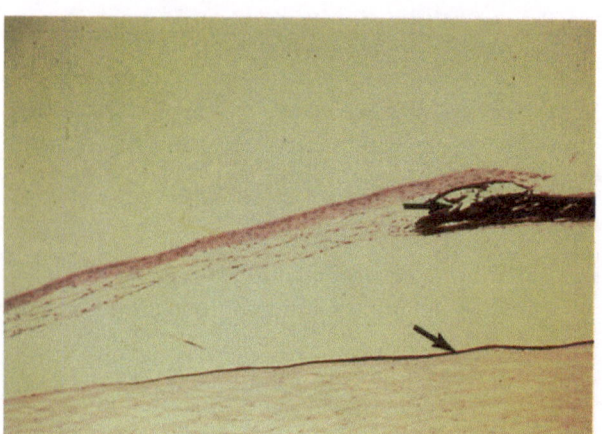

FIGURE 2-8.
Photomicrograph demonstrating calcium in the cornea of a patient with band keratopathy. (Von Kossa stain) (arrows)

FIGURE 2-9.
Polymorphonuclear leukocytes in a patient with pars planitis. (H & E)

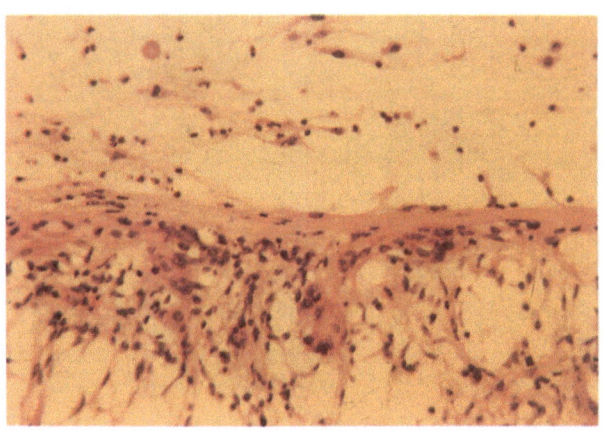

FIGURE 2-10.
Eosinophil in vitreous from a patient with *Toxocara canis.* (H & E)

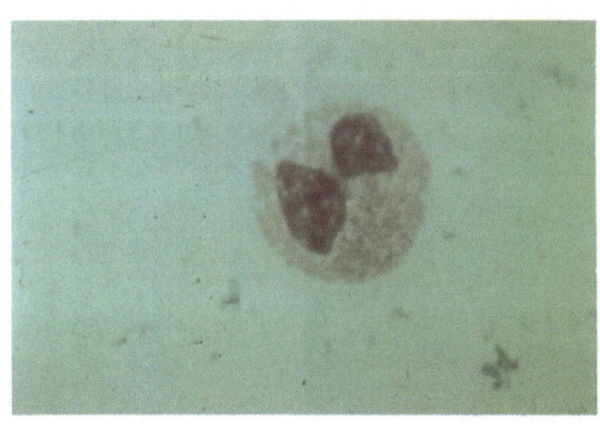

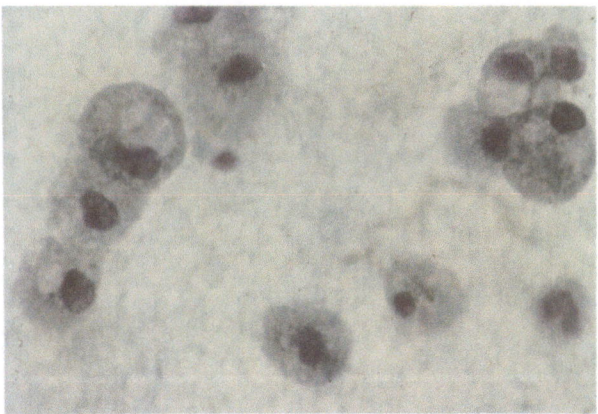

FIGURE 2-11.
These macrophages were present in a tap from a patient with phacolytic glaucoma. (Giemsa)

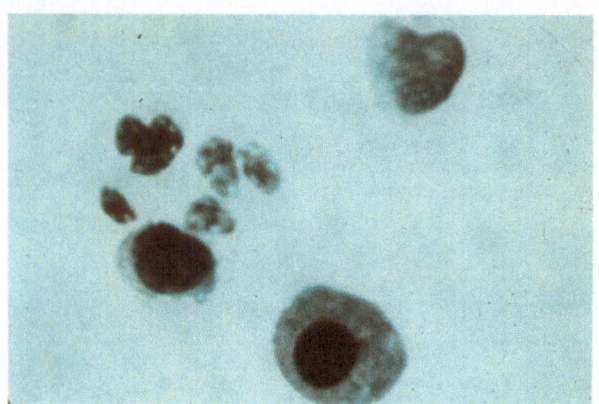

FIGURE 2-12.
Plasma cell. (Peroxidase)

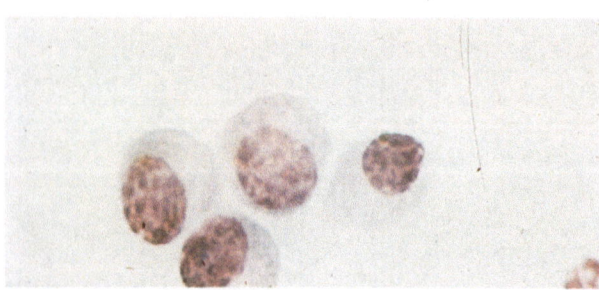

FIGURE 2-13.
Lymphocyte. (H & E)

Chapter 3

Basics of Ocular Genetics

The adage "like father like son" and some friend's comment that you are a "clone" of one of your parents introduces us to the concept of genetics. Why do we have our father's eyes or our mother's nose? The answer lies in our chromosomes. Our 46 chromosomes are two sets of 23 chromosomes derived from each parent. One member of each 23 chromosomal pairs is inherited from the father and the other from the mother. Via this method the child has half the genetic material from each parent. The total of 46 chromosomes includes two that determine the sex of the child. An XX determines a female, and the XY pair denotes a male.

With this simplistic overview of who we are, some of the basic concepts of genetics and how they apply to ophthalmology are presented. The genetic information coded by each chromosome is carried on its genes. The genes code for a specific protein, which in turn is pooled with all the other proteins made by other genes on that or other chromosomes. The result is the myriad information that makes up a human being. If an abnormality occurs in the gene, an altered product is the result. If that protein is insignificant, the organism does not manifest that abnormality. If, on the other hand, that protein was essential, the organism shows evidence of that abnormality. A good example is the substitution of one amino acid ultimately producing a disease called sickle cell anemia. It must be remembered that some mutations must be on both pairs of the chromosome to be clinically evident. If only one of the chromosomes carries the defect, the organism may be a carrier for that defect. Possessing only half the total information for the product may not result in clinical disease, as 50% of the protein may be enough for the organism to function well. The decreased amount of enzyme or protein might not be known unless a specific assay for that enzyme or protein is performed to quantitate its amount. The defect does not become evident unless that individual mates with someone who is also a carrier. Their child, then, may have the defect on both chromosomes (a 1:4 chance) and thus exhibit the mutation clinically. This type of inheritance is called autosomal recessive (Table 3-1). If the abnormal protein is essential and is present on one of the two chromosomes, the organism would exhibit the abnormality, which defines autosomal dominant inheritance (Table 3-2). If the abnormalities are present on the X chromosome, we can then speak of sex (or X)-linked dominant (Table 3-3) or X-linked recessive (Table 3-4) traits. Because the female has two X chromosomes, the normal X balances the abnormal X, and that female phenotypically appears normal. If she passes on the abnormal X to her son, the child will have the condition. Her daughter, on the other hand, would be

TABLE 3-1.
Common Characteristics of Autosomal Recessive Inheritance

Abnormal gene does not produce clinical disease
Double dose of abnormal gene produces clinical disease
Male/female ratio = 1:1
Each child has a 1:4 chance of being affected
Consanguinity is common

TABLE 3-2.
Common Characteristics of Autosomal Dominant Transmission

Vertical transmission of the defect
Affected individual usually has an affected parent
Male/female ratio = 1:1
Unaffected persons do not transmit the trait
Generally these entities are milder

TABLE 3-3.
Characteristics of Sex-Linked (X-Linked) Dominant Inheritance

Both males and females affected
Trait is twice as frequent in females unless the trait is fatal in males
Affected males transmit disease to all daughters but not to sons
Affected females transmit to daughters and sons equally

TABLE 3-4.
Common Characteristics of Sex-Linked (X-Linked) Recessive Inheritance

Males predominantly affected
Affected males have carrier daughters
Affected males related to carrier female
Affected males who marry carriers have 50% affected daughters and
           50% carrier daughters
Absence of father to son transmission

similar to the mother. Thus the carrier mother passes the abnormal gene to 50% of her offspring. One-half the girls would be carriers and one-half of the boys would be affected.

There is also a group of inherited diseases that do not conform to our traditional patterns of inheritance. Maternal inheritance through mitochondrial DNA describes a group of diseases such as Leber's hereditary optic neuropathy, ragged red fiber disease, and inherited myoclonus epilepsy.

There are many times when we are sure an individual has a particular gene. For example, the patient's parents are normal, but the grandparents exhibit the same condition as the patient. This phenomenon can be explained by penetrance. The normal appearing parent may actually have the abnormality but it is not exhibited phenotypically. The gene may even express itself to varying degrees within the same family. All family members do not have every hallmark sign of a specific disease. Associated with this concept is the notion that certain aspects of the disease appear at certain times. The Marfan syndrome patient may have long fingers and be tall as a child but might not develop an aortic aneurysm until the third decade of life.

Other phenotypical abnormalities may be the product of portions of a chromosome being deleted, shuffled to a new location (translocation), or even duplicating itself. On occasion the entire chromosome may duplicate itself, resulting in a trisomy condition (e.g., trisomy 21, or Down syndrome).

Although a trait may be dominant in its genetic transmission, it may produce only one defect. On the other hand, one gene may code for a defect that manifests in many systems, that is, it is pleotropic.

Genetic counseling becomes an important part of ophthalmology because many ocular disorders have genetic aspects. For example, the parents of a child with retinoblastoma want to know whether they will have more affected children. The answer to such a question is not easy unless the ophthalmologist has done his or her homework. The physician must first make an accurate diagnosis, as the counseling is based on a certain entity and its genetic mode of transmission. That being established, the ophthalmologist must sleuth the family history. It is not enough to casually inquire about grandparents. Detailed information must be sought, such as consanguinity, adoption, whether the current parents are the biological parents of the child, and the health histories of all family members. Some conditions will not be known as a separate entity by the patient. If the patient has angioid streaks, however, we might not be able to elicit a history that someone else had angioid streaks. The ophthalmologist then might have to inquire about family members being able to bend their fingers excessively or someone having excessive laxed skin around their neck.

Ophthalmologists should be aware of the genetic and clinical facets of the disorder, as they must inform the parents or patient of what the defect means in terms of function, morbidity, and mortality. The ophthalmologist is merely an informer; and if the counseling is successful, the parents make their own decisions about the next child. Some families opt to have more children despite the high risk or the ultimate fate of those children. They may want to know whether amniocentesis would be of any benefit. If the ophthalmologist cannot answer their questions, a geneticist may be able to complete the counseling for the parents.

Selected Reading

Apple DJ (1974). Chromosome-induced Ocular Disease in Goldberg MF (editor): Genetic and Metabolic Eye Disease. Boston: Little, Brown & Co.

Gelehter TD, Collins FS (1990). Principles of Medical Genetics. Baltimore: Williams & Wilkins

Musarella MA (1992). Gene mapping of ocular diseases. Surv Ophthalmol 36:285-312

Chapter 4

Methods of Examination

Ophthalmologists were students of medicine or osteopathy before entering their subspecialty. The ocular examination begins by focusing on the entire patient, which takes advantage of the ophthalmologist's full medical knowledge. There is no excuse for omitting the basics such as a good history of present illness, medical history, ocular history, review of systems, medications, and allergies. This general inquiry is then followed by a complete ocular examination.

During our era of medicolegal confrontations, the possibility of lawsuits is always present and so other details should be kept in mind as well. The patient's complete name should be documented as well as aliases or variations he or she might use. This information facilitates record keeping and ensures that the correct patient is identified. Addresses, telephone numbers, and any data pertaining to compensation must be recorded. It is well to keep in mind that nothing the patient says is too trivial to document. It may be a stray comment that alerts you to possible future problems.

Determination of the patient's medical history is paramount. Specific questions relating to each organ system must be asked. Patients do not understand esoteric medical terms. Common terms are often used to describe a disease entity, such as "bad blood," which is a street term for syphilis. On occasion the patient heard the medical term for the disease but did not listen. The patient may not consider eyedrops to be medication because they are only drops. Specific questions about prematurity, childhood diseases, and surgeries should be elicited from the patient, or in the case of a child, from the parent.

An ophthalmic history of the present illness should be documented chronologically. If the patient is a child, record both the child's and the parent's versions. Associated symptoms such as bumping into things at night or during the daylight hours may serve as clues to the diagnosis of the patient's condition. If anyone accompanies the patient, he or she should be listed on the record. Although patients often insist that they were never told anything by the last ophthalmologist they saw, the accompanying member may shed some alternate light on the subject. Often it is necessary to call that physician to find out what the patient was told, if the physician referred the patient, and (if so) why the patient was referred.

Examination

Visual acuity should be the first determination, as it is an excellent determiner of visual function. The acuity should be documented with and without the best correction. A pinhole acuity test can determine the patient's best possible acuity. Near vision is noted with Jaeger or point notation and at the distance used by the patient. Although we commonly measure near vision at 14 inches, many patients read at other distances. The patient must not be allowed to determine the end of the visual acuity test but should be pushed to guess the letters or numbers on increasingly smaller lines. The examiner then decides when a sufficient number of errors have been made, and the best acuity is determined.

Visual acuity determinations in infants and children may be somewhat more difficult. The acuity determination should be performed as accurately as possible, as it may determine the child's future development. An undiagnosed and easily treatable visual disorder can set up a cascade of adverse sequences that may deprive the child of his or her early learning experiences. There are practical clues to the visual status of the child. For toddlers, begin by observing the children. Do they look around the room? If there is something within their reach, do they attempt to touch it? If the mother walks away, can the child find her without her calling? Children's innate reaction to light is another method for determining if they see light. Infants turn toward a diffuse light. If you place the light 180 degrees from its original orientation, normal children turn their heads toward the new direction of light. In toddlers over the age of 5 months, the ophthalmologist can use the blinking response to a threatening gesture. The tester must be sure that the draft created by the tester is not the stimulus to which the child reacts. Finally, children can be assessed by their ability to fixate on an object. The object should be large enough and quiet, so only the ability to fix is tested. (Fig. 4-1). Infants can be assessed by whether they reach for an object. We find that this method is a good way to test infants over 6 months of age.

Much has been written about contrast sensitivity testing being used as an adjunct to visual acuity testing. There are several acquired conditions, such as glaucoma, diabetic retinopathy, and amblyopia, in which there is a definite loss of contrast sensitivity although near-normal visual acuity is maintained. Although traditional contrast testing requires expensive and sophisticated techniques, there are some easily performed clinical methods that work. Arden plates and the Visitech Vision Contrast Test System, the Regan Letter Chart, and the Pelli-Robson letter chart are but a few.

The potential acuity meter (PAM) projects a small Snellen chart through lenticular opacities to predict the best possible visual acuity in that patient. False-negative and-false positive results sometimes can be a problem with this and other tools such as a laser interferometer.

Much has been written about the use of optokinetic nystagmus (OKN) as a reliable indicator of a child's visual acuity. Although it is absent in blind infants, several variables accompany the test for OKN. The child must be attentive and should have intact motor responses. Testing a child with a drum from a 3-foot distance may reveal that the child is more interested in the tester than in the drum. If the child is held facing the examiner and rotated, nystagmus occurs. It is dampened if the child focuses on the examiner but occurs as the child is rotated. When the movement is stopped, the child should show a few beats of nystagmus. An absent OKN in a non seizing child indicates a poor acuity.

Electrophysiological testing such as an electroretinogram (ERG) and visual evoked cortical potentials (VECP) may be useful in children and adults. Visual evoked potentials (VEPs), another term for VECP, can be elicited by either a pattern stimulus or a flash stimulus. Pattern responses are superior in that the waveform and latency are better visualized and developed; however, infants and toddlers must be attentive in order to demonstrate waveforms reliably. (Figs. 4-2 and 4-3). The light stimulus, or more recently the diode pattern stimulus, works well with infants and toddlers. We find that a hungry (not famished) child takes a bottle quietly and allows the examiner to put on electrodes for either ERG or VEP testing. It is important to remember that an ERG is a mass response, and a child with no macular vision has a normal ERG. Further testing with VEPs may indicate that there is a lesion in the optic pathway.

Gross examination is important, as observation of the patient often provides clues to the problem. In cases of congenital anomaly, it is wise to open the infant's mouth and observe the palate. Moreover, some anomalies are associated with low-set ears or certain body characteristics (e.g., a webbed neck in Turner Syndrome). The whole patient must be examined before we devote the rest of our time to the ocular system.

The child or adult should be tested for a Marcus-Gunn pupil; if present, it indicates an afferent pupillary defect. On occasion, a reverse Marcus-Gunn pupil is seen.

The ocular ductions and versions should be examined. Esotropia may be a clue that a retinoblastoma lurks in a child. A child with sunset eyes could be harboring a pinealoma or a problem in the fourth ventricle.

The anterior segment is usually evaluated with a slit lamp. The cornea, anterior chamber, iris, and lens should be scrutinized for any suggestion of associated congenital lesions (Fig. 4-4). In infants and premature neonates in the nursery, we use a 20-diopter lens as a magnifier to study the anterior segment. In adults the lens should be evaluated for signs of congenital cataracts, e.g., sutural, cerulean, or polar (Fig. 4-5). Pupillary membranes or fibrils are the remnants of the once present tunica vasculosa lentis.

The examiner should use low power on the slit lamp to obtain a better panoramic view of the eye. For example, having the patient look up and then down demonstrates whether the vitreous is detached; if detached it sweeps up and then down. The examiner can also determine from the slit lamp examination if there are vitreous membranes in the patient with an optically empty vitreous, suggesting a vitreoretinal degeneration, such as with Wagner or Stickler syndrome. In adults, while the patient is at the slit lamp, a 60- or 90-diopter lens or a Hruby lens can be placed in front of the eye to obtain a panoramic view of the posterior pole (Fig. 4-6). Finally, a Zeiss prism lens is adequate for evaluting the anterior chamber angles.

The pupils are dilated with tropicamide (Mydriacyl) 1% (or 0.5% if mini-

mal dilation is needed) and 2.5% phenylephrine. We avoid 10% phenylephrine because it raises blood pressure in children and adults. We also avoid
cyclopentolate (particularly 2%) in infants and premature neonates because
it can produce seizures. Always inform the parents that the child will be
sleepy after the dilation drops have taken effect. Some parents even ask
where they can get "some of those drops"! Do not forget that tropicamide
stings, which in children can be a major problem. Giving a topical anesthet-
ic before the dilating drops facilitates the dilation process. We find that
telling the child it will hurt is far better, as they then later believe and trust
you. Telling them that the drops do not hurt and then having them sur-
prised by the stinging is far more devastating and sets a bad tone for the
rest of the visit.

When the patient's pupils have dilated, it is time to evaluate the fundus.
Direct ophthalmoscopy is done initially to obtain an overall view. The optic
nerve and macula can be examined to rule out anomalies. There are problems with the limited field size (10 degrees), depth of field, and magnification (15x). The patient must not make roving eye movements or have a
high refractive/astigmatic error or hazy media, as either would interfere
with a good view of the posterior pole.

The indirect lens and indirect ophthalmoscope are necessary tools for
examining the fundus. Magnification can be obtained using a 14-diopter
lens (4x), which enables the examiner to see the entire posterior pole with
some magnification. The 20-diopter lens magnifies 3.5x and a 30- diopter
lens 2x. The 30-diopter lens provides the examiner with a panoramic view.
Relations between structures can be better appreciated when anatomical
locations can be discerned. In children, a wide view of the fundus provides
more information in less time than when examining the child with the 20-
diopter lens. Because of its greater field, the 30-diopter lens is excellent for
examining children in the nurseries. It affords the best view of the fundus
in situations where there is little room to move around the patient.

The adult patient should be examined lying on a table or in a chair that
is capable of converting to a table. The drawing pad is placed on the
patient's chest, and the examiner begins to sketch the fundus (Fig. 4-7). It
is well to follow a logical order. We prefer to begin with the disc, vasculature, and macula in one eye and thereafter sketch the two nasal quadrants
and the two temporal quadrants. Attention is then turned to the other eye,
drawing its parts in the same order.

Indirect ophthalmoscopy in children may be difficult. For the unsedated
child, wrapping the child in a sheet with the parent holding the child's head
and an assistant holding the child's body or legs allows examination. A
"papoose" is another technique used to restrain children.

We prefer not to wear a white jacket when we see children. White jackets
have a bad connotation, and often the examination must be cut short
because the child is screaming in fear of a possible needlestick.

The rheostat is left on low to acclimate the patient's eye to the bright
lights. The illumination is slowly increased until the examiner is able to illu-
minate the fundus adequately. It is not good practice to turn the illumination to its highest level, as it hurts the patient and, with children, abruptly
ends the examination.

Part of the funduscopic evaluation is scleral indentation (depression). It
is an art to indent the periphery in a patient without eliciting squeals of

pain and, on occasion, expletives. The examiner must be gentle so the patient does not fear an injury to the eye. The indentation is applied tangentially after the end of the indentor is apposed on the lids (Fig. 4-8). Little force is needed to adequately depress and produce a mound on the retina. If too much force is used, the mound becomes so large the examiner does not appreciate it and presses even more. It is important that there is one plane between the examiner's eyes, the lens, the patient's pupil, and the patient's retina, ensuring that the examiner can see the image. To examine the patient's 12 o'clock region, the examiner must observe from below with the scleral indentor at the 12 o'clock position and the patient looking superiorly. The opposite is true when examining the 6 o'clock position.

A Goldmann three-mirror lens is used to obtain a virtual erect image of the fundus (Fig. 4-9). The periphery can be examined using one of the mirrors, thus giving the examiner information on peripheral retinal relations and pathological details. The images seen in the mirrors are located 180 degrees opposite to the lesion in the mirror. The images are not crossed in the mirrors. The examiner should begin with the central view, examining the retrolental space and anterior vitreous. Thereafter the examiner must observe the remainder of the vitreous, looking for membranes, cells, or any other anatomical deviation from normal. The disc vessels and macula are seen last. The mirrors are then utilized to see the equatorial and peripheral structures. Children do not usually enjoy having a lens placed on their eye, and it may have to be done in the operating room using an operating microscope using the same sequence as described above for adults. Other lenses such as the Mainster, Panfunduscope, or Volk's equatorial lenses can be utilized diagnostically (Fig. 4-10).

There are times when the child cannot be easily examined in the office despite sedation with chloral hydrate. These children must undergo general anesthesia for a complete funduscopic evaluation. Usually, ketamine or nitrous oxide are used for these procedures.

Additional Testing

Potential Acuity Measurement

The potential acuity test projects light onto the patient's macula. The machine projects increasingly smaller numbers or letters onto the fovea to determine the macula's best possible acuity.

Color Vision Testing

Objects in our world truly do not possess color but reflect the more than 8 million shades and tints our complex visual system can impart on them. The clinical evaluation of color vision is based on identifying an abnormality in color matching and chromatic discrimination. Simple testing for congenital color vision abnomalities requires the Ishihara or A-O Hardy-Rand-Rittler plates. These tests detect congenital red-green color deficiencies when placed at a distance of 75 cm from the patient. The Farnsworth-Munsell 100 hue and Farnsworth panel (D-15) tests are much more sophisticated and are suited for elucidating tritan defects and acquired loss of color vision. The Nagel anomaloscope and the Sloan acromatopsia test are other methods for evaluating the color system in humans.

Ultrasonography

The use of ultrasonography has allowed us to enter a new diagnostic era in ophthalmology (Table 4-1; Fig. 4-11). It is no longer necessary to guess when an accurate picture of the internal structures is possible; ultrasonography allows the examiner to evaluate both anterior and posterior structures with a high degree of accuracy. The posterior segment is best examined using a contact method; and the anterior segment is best visualized by immersion techniques. Positioning the patient begins the examination. The machine must be placed near the head of the patient so the probe can be easily manipulated while the examiner looks at the screen (Fig. 4-12). The trigger used to freeze the scan should be readily available.

Scanning must be done in the horizontal and vertical directions to obtain a complete picture of the eye. The vertical scans are midline vertical, vertical nasotemporal, and vertical temporonasal. Likewise, the horizontal planes are midline horizontal, horizontal superoinferior, and horizontal inferosuperior. These six meridians represent the minimum number of planes that must be scanned to obtain a reliable picture of the intraocular structures.

After all the scans have been made, a composite drawing should be done that encompasses all the views obtained. The physician should perform the scan, not a technician. Ultrasonography is a dynamic tool that is interpreted as the test is performed. Having a physician interpret a scan that has been done by someone else can lead to erroneous conclusions.

TABLE 4-1.
Indications for Ultrasonography

Opacity of ocular structures
      Corneal opacification
      Hyphema
      Hypopyon/intraocular inflammation
      Pupillary membrane
      Cataract
      Persistent primary hyperplastic vitreous (PHPV)
      Retinopathy of prematurity
      Vitreous hemorrhage

Tumors
      Retinoblastoma

Miscellaneous lesions
      Retinal detachment: exudative/rhegmatogenous
      Optic disc anomalies

Simultaneous A-scan recordings are obtained to confirm what is seen on the B-scan. It allows the examiner to differentiate between tissue densities for purposes of comparison.

Visual Fields Tests

Confrontation visual fields tests can be easily performed on most adults and children. It is a simple, unsophisticated way of determining the extent of panorama seen by the patient. More sophisticated testing requires a tangent screen, Goldmann perimeter, or automated perimeter.

Fluorescein Angiography

Fluorescein angiography involves injection of sodium fluorescein, which when exposed to excitation and barrier filters presents a dynamic view of the ocular circulation within 8-15 seconds after it has been injected into a peripheral vein. Ordinarily, if the tight junctions between adjacent retinal pigment epithelial cells and capillary endothelial cells are intact, the fluorescein molecules do not pass out of the circulation.

After fluorescein is injected into a vein, it first appears in the choroid, producing a choroidal flush. One to two seconds later it enters the central retinal artery and retinal arterioles. After passing through the arterioles it traverses the capillaries, the venules, the veins, and finally the central retinal vein. The *term laminar* flow is used to describe the phenomenon of fluorescence along the sides of the venules and veins while the faster central lumen is dark. As more and more fluorescein enters the veins, the entire lumen fluoresces. Cilioretinal vessels fill with the choroid, whereas the disc fluoresces from branches of the central retinal artery and the posterior ciliary circulation. Abnormalities are diagnosed if there is hypo- or hyperfluorescence when neither is expected (Figs. 4-13 and 4-14). There are many causes of fluorescein blockage, for example, exudates (hard and soft), blood, tumors, melanin, lipofucsin, edema of the pigment epithelium, foreign bodies, and nonperfusion. The macula is normally hypofluorescent owing to xanthophyll pigment. Leakage or pooling of the fluorescein produces hyperfluorescence. It is also possible that structures within the eye appear to fluoresce with the administration of any fluorescein to the patient; this phenomenon is called *pseudofluorescence*. It is also important to observe for symmetrical filling of the vessels in the superior and inferior retinas.

Electrophysiology

Dark Adaptation

We all experience a few moments of dark vision as we enter a dark room, such as a theater. After a few moments of adapting to the dark, we can easily find our seats. What of the patient who after 10-20 minutes still cannot tell if there are any empty seats? The response to dark-adaptation testing involves a rod component and a cone component. Typically, the curve demonstrates the cone threshold, the cone-rod break, and finally the rod threshold. The recovery time for cones after exposure to a bright light is 10 minutes, and the rod recovery time is 50 minutes. Although cones recover faster, the level of sensitivity is greater in the rods.

Electroretinogram/Electrooculogram

The electroretinogram (ERG) represents a mass electrical response of the retina to a light stimulus. The response waveform is composed of several retinal structures (Fig. 4-15). The cone density is maximal in the fovea (central 5 degrees) whereas the rod density is maximal 20-40 degrees eccentric to the fovea. More than 90% of the cones lie outside the fovea, yet the numbers of rods and cones within the macula are comparable.

We can monitor the functional state of the rods and cones, (i.e., the photoreceptors) by obtaining an ERG. The ERG is composed of various parts. The initial negative deflection originates from the photoreceptors, the a-wave. The b-wave, which follows the a-wave, originates from Müller cells. Repolarization, or the c-wave, is a function of the pigment epithelium. The early receptor potential (ERP) is seen on the ascending limb of the b-wave and originates from the photoreceptor outer segments. There are other minor components of the ERG, such as the d-wave, oscillatory potentials, and w-waves.

Electroretinographic testing is useful for detecting or confirming hereditary retinal degenerations. The ERG can be subnormal or even abnormal years before an ophthalmologist detects clinical signs of disease in the fundus. The ERG can be also used to differentiate juvenile macular degeneration (normal ERG) from cone-rod degeneration (abnormal ERG). Patients in whom Refsum's or Bassen-Kornzweig syndrome is suspected have an abnormal ERG along with abnormal phytanic acid levels and serum β-lipoprotein (abetalipoproteinemia).

We can influence the magnitude of the ERG response by varying the dark adaptation of the patient or the background illumination. Characteristically, the response is obtained by placing a contact lens on the cornea of a dilated patient. The grounded patient has a reference electrode placed at the temples and is seated at a Ganzfield stimulus. Cone function is exemplified by testing photopically with bright white light. Dim white light or a blue light brings out the rod response. Rods and cones both react to red light. The flicker fusion records the response to increasing frequency of light flashes. It distinguishes cone activity from rod activity. Higher frequencies allow the rod response to drop out. Table 4-2 lists some of the conditions for which an ERG helps make or confirm the diagnosis.

It is not possible to seat infants at a Ganzfield apparatus and apply corneal electodes, much less a corneal contact lens. In some cases, sedation with chloral hydrate at 20-40 mg/kg/24 hours permits electrophysiological testing. We have found that a hungry child is more interested in food than electrodes. Patience with the child and parent is often an indispensible tool when performing such tests on children. In infants or in the nursery, an ERG is done with a timing light, which produces a recordable response. (Fig. 4-16).

TABLE 4-2.
Retinal /Choroidal Diseases that Produce an Abnormal ERG

Congenital stationary night blindness
Retinitis pigmentosa
Leber's congenital amaurosis
Gyrate atrophy
Choroideremia
Rod-cone degeneration
Color blindness
Toxic amblyopia
Siderosis
Vitamin deficiency
Nutritional deficiency
Occlusive vascular disorders

The electrooculogram (EOG) is a less used measurement of retinal function. Principally testing the pigment epithelium, it produces a response based on the fact that the eye is a dipole with the cornea being positive and the retina negative. As the eye moves left and right, the pigment epithelium generates the potential. The potentials are measured in both the light- and dark-adapted states. The potentials elicited by the light phase of the testing period are divided by the potentials seen during the dark phase of the testing period and a value obtained. Values above 1.85 are normal whereas values below 1.85 are abnormal. Table 4-3 lists some of the conditions for which an abnormal EOG is to be expected.

Visual Evoked Cortical Responses

The VECP, also known as the VEP, reflects the integrity of the visual paths from the fovea through the optic nerve throught the geniculate bodies to the occipital cortex. Primarily, the test uses a light stimulus or an alternating checkerboard stimulus. Light emission diodes (LED) goggles can be used in infants (Fig. 4-17).

TABLE 4-3.
Indications for an EOG

Best's disease
Leber's congenital amaurosis
Retinitis albipuctata
Retinitis punctata albescens
Pattern dystrophy of the reginal pigment epithelium
Dominant drusen
Ocular albinism
Stargardt's disease
Rod-cone degeneration
Fundus flavimaculatus
Chloroquine retinopathy

TABLE 4-4.
Electrophysiological Tests

Disorder	VECP	ERG	EOG
Macular disease	Abnormal	Normal	Normal (Except in Best's disease)
Optic nerve disease	Abnormal	Normal	Normal
Hysteria	Normal	Normal	Normal

Often a child is referred for an evaluation. Because the eyes react involuntarily, the examiner can easily obtain information as to the status of the optic nerve and macula, especially when the fundi appear normal. Combined use of these electrophysiological tests can often separate hysteria from optic nerve/macula disease (Table 4-4).

Summary

The ophthalmologist now has the tools required to assess the visual system in the office setting. Hospital ancillary testing, such as with computed tomography or magnetic resonance imaging, can also be helpful. These sophisticated and expensive tests are not, however, a substitute for a good history and physical examination.

Selected Reading

Hart Jr WM (ed) (1992). Adler's Physiology of the Eye. Clinical Application. 9th Ed. St Louis: Mosby-Year Book

Huismans H (Tetz MR, Apple DJ, translators) (1990). The Ocular Fundus. Baltimore: Williams & Wilkins

Krill AE (1977). Hereditary Retinal and Choroidal Diseases. Vols. 1 and 2. Hagerstown, MD: Harper & Row

Mets MB, Maumenee IH (1983). The eye and the chromosome. Surv Ophthalmol 28:20-32

Ryan SJ (ed) (1989). Retina. St. Louis: Mosby

Spencer WH, Font RL, Green WR, et al (eds) (1985). Ophthalmic Pathology. An Atlas and Textbook. 3rd Ed. Philadelphia: Saunders

Figures

FIGURE 4-1.
(A) Stuffed toy that does not make any noise and is either yellow or red is a good fixation object. The child sees the object and smiles. If the object is moved around, the child should be able to follow it. (B) Toddlers also follow a bright object.

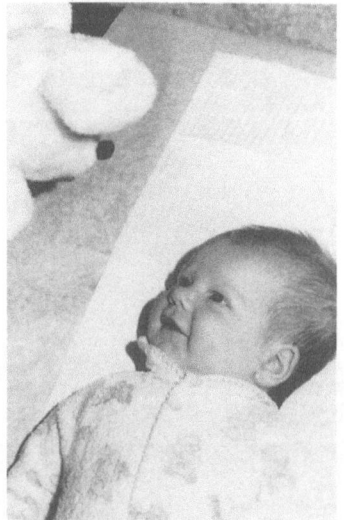

A

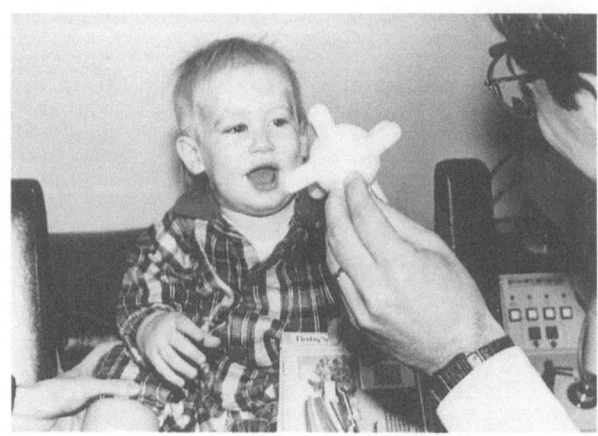

B

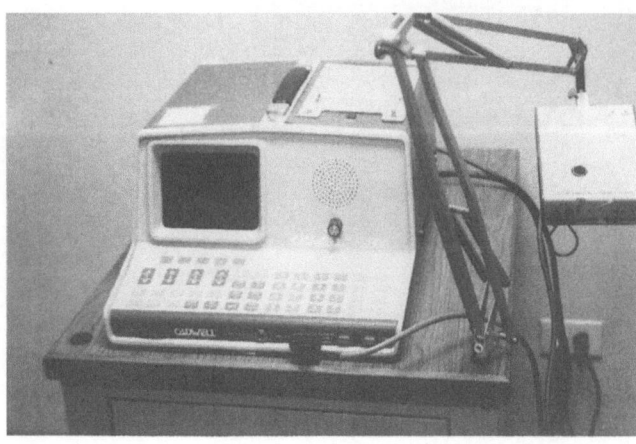

FIGURE 4-2.
We prefer to use a Cadwell machine, as it is small and portable. Electrophysiological testing can be done in the operating room under anesthesia with little difficulty.

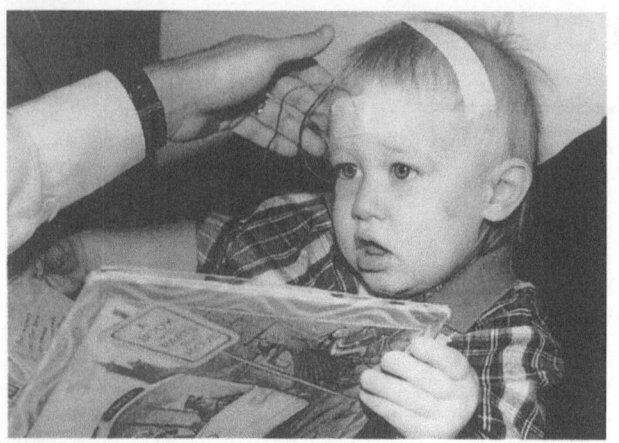

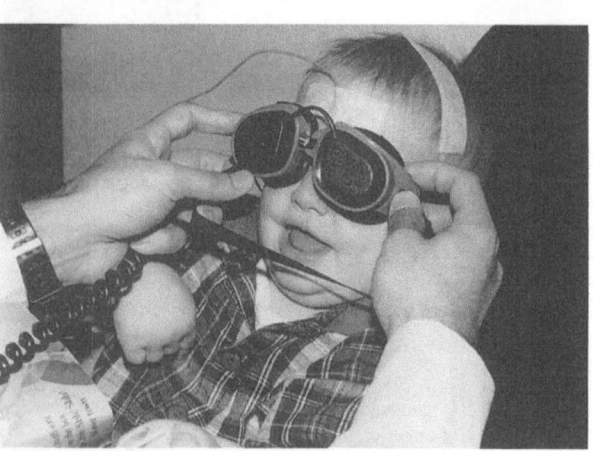

FIGURE 4-3.
(A) If the child is kept occupied with a stuffed toy or picture book, the electrodes can be placed in preparation for an ERG or VECP. (B) Use of the LED goggles is easy with toddlers. This little fellow thinks the red lights are funny. In no time a complete VECP can be performed.

A

B

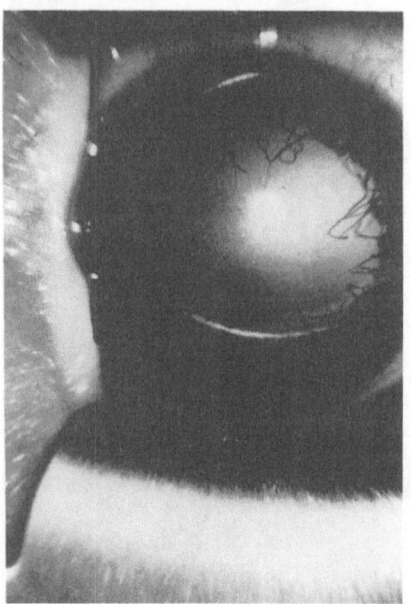

FIGURE 4-4.
Anterior segment should be evaluated. Congenital anterior segment entities, such as pupillary remnants in older children or a persistent tunica vasculosa lentis, as in this case, become evident.

FIGURE 4-5.

This young man has several anomalies, including an iris coloboma that opens in the inferonasal quadrant, respecting the fetal fissure. If you observe the lens, you can see that the embryonal nucleus has an opacity as well as a polar cataract.

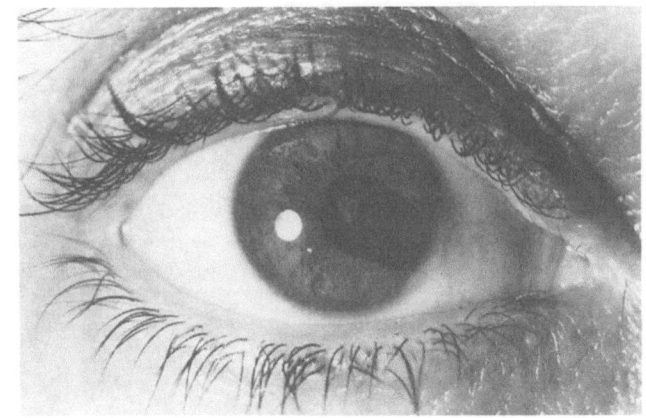

FIGURE 4-6.

Previously a Hruby lens was standard issue on slit lamp biomicroscopes. Even easier to use is the 60- or 90-diopter lens. The 60-diopter lens (left) provides a more panoramic view of the posterior pole out toward the equator. The 90-diopter lens (right) is excellent for an in-depth study of foveal tissues.

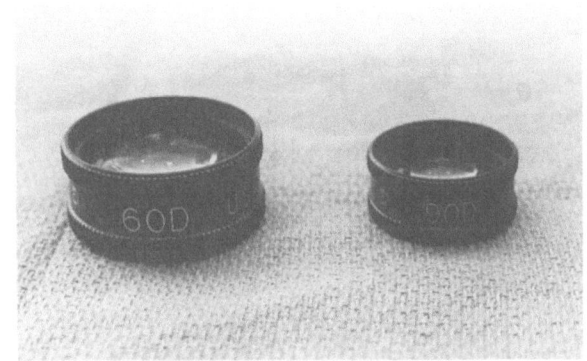

FIGURE 4-7.

The fundus should be drawn. Photography is convenient, but many abnormalities cannot be appreciated. Drawing forces the examiner to study the patient's retina. With the patient in the reclining position, examiners can easily position themselves and sketch the retina in as much detail as possible. The examiner places the drawing pad on the patient's chest upside down so it matches the image seen in the lens. Upon rotating the pad, the sketch anatomically correlates with the patient's fundus.

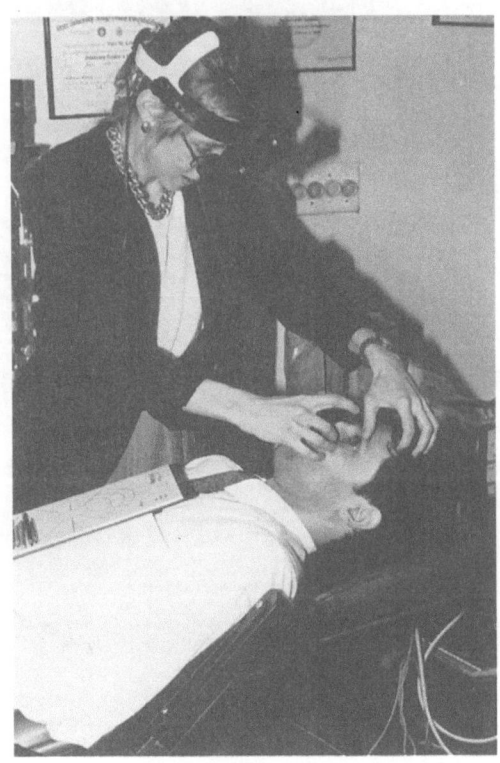

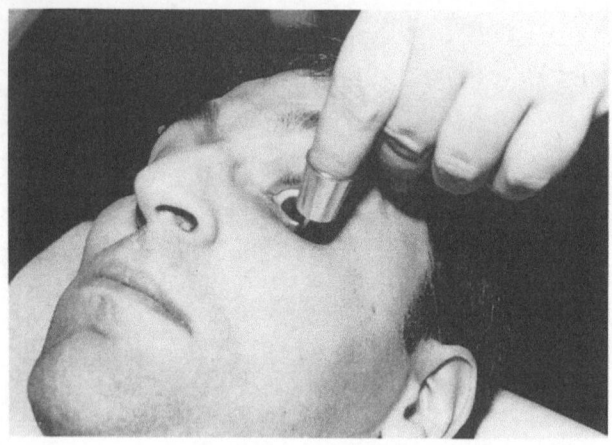

FIGURE 4-8.
Indentors need only be placed at the lid margin. The patient is asked to look in that direction, which should be enough to produce a scleral mound. Too much pressure makes too large a mound, which is not appreciated in the lens (or by the patient).

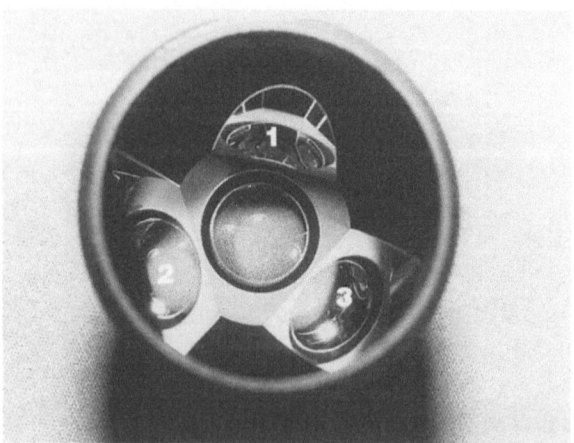

FIGURE 4-9.
When using the Goldmann three-mirror lens, the examiner should be aware of what can be examined. The central area enables the examiner to view the posterior pole. The smallest mirror (1) enables the examiner to view the angles and, in an aphakic, well-dilated eye, the pars plana. The trapezoidal mirror (2) permits the area from the arcades to just past the equator to be visualized. The rectangular mirror (3) permits the periphery to be examined.

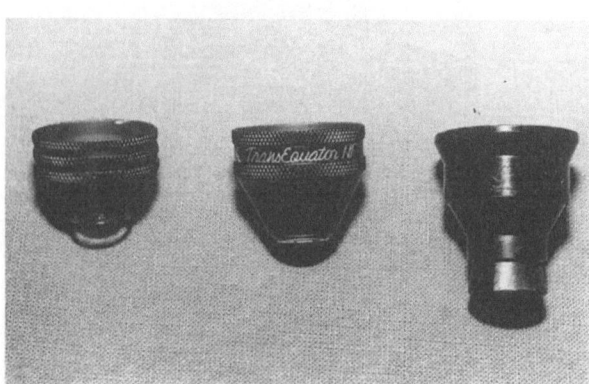

FIGURE 4-10.
Fundus lenses that can be used to examine the fundus (and photocoagulate it). They essentially are indirect lenses that are placed on the cornea and allow the examiner to see beyond the equator. From left: Volk's Panfunduscope; Volk's Transequatorial No-Fluid; Rodenstock's Panfunduscope.

FIGURE 4-11.
Ultrasonography is important. B-scans provide much information if physicians who request the examination perform it themselves. Machines displaying simultaneous A- and B-scans are preferable.

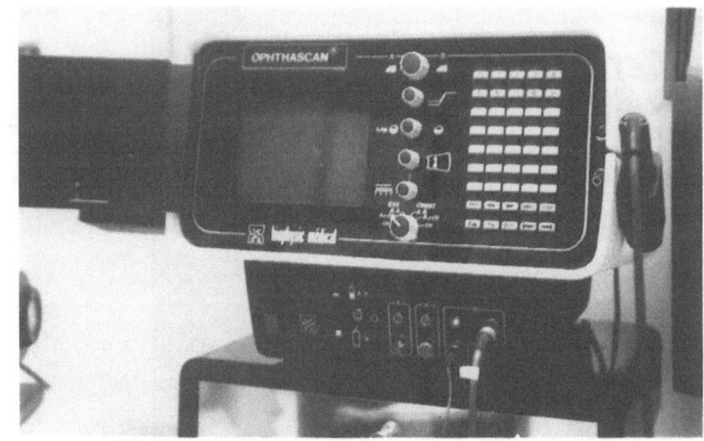

FIGURE 4-12.
Be sure to touch the child's arm with the ultrasound probe before placing it on the lids. If the child is otherwise engaged, the process can be done quickly and without trauma to child or physician.

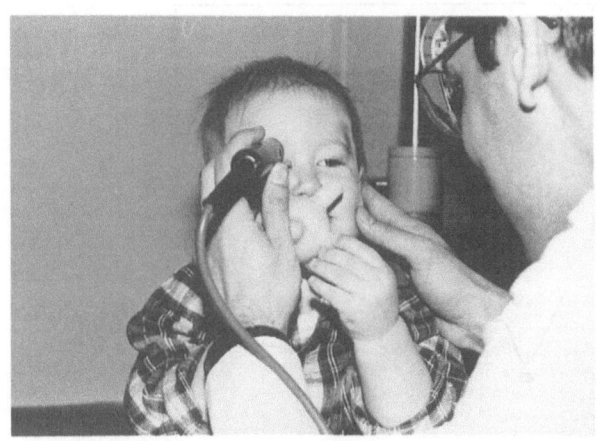

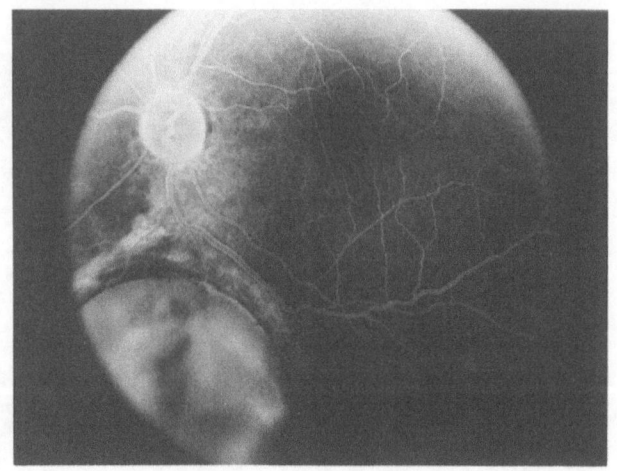

FIGURE 4-13.
Angiogram showing fluorescence around the edge of a retinal coloboma. The apparent fluorescence of the coloboma itself corresponds to the sclera. Hypofluorescence is seen at the fovea. The vasculature fills more in the superior retina than it does in the inferior retina.

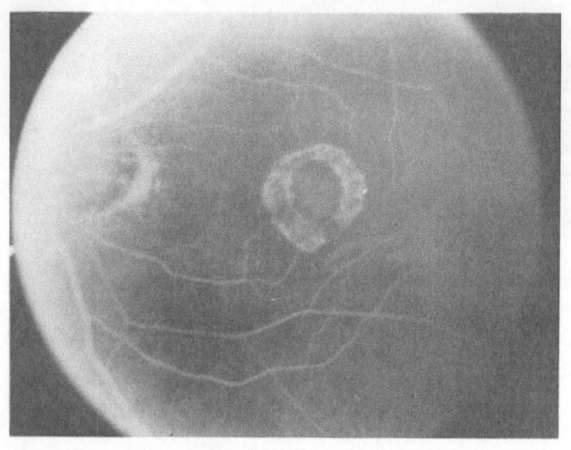

FIGURE 4-14.
Angiogram showing hypofluorescence at the macula with a surrounding hypopigmented ring—halo nevus. The arteries and veins are both filled with fluorescein.

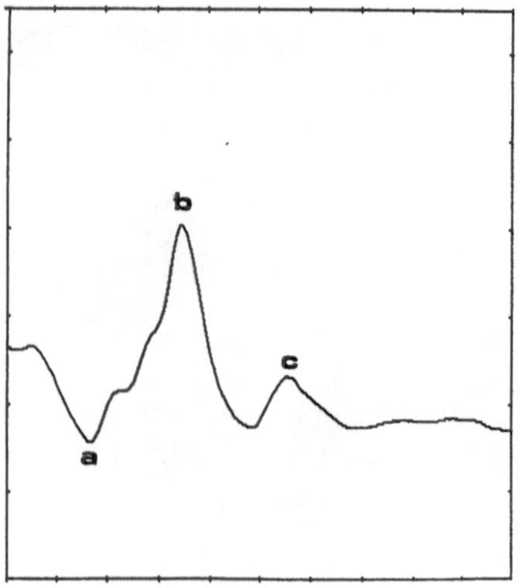

FIGURE 4-15.
Typical electroretinogram with indicated waves.

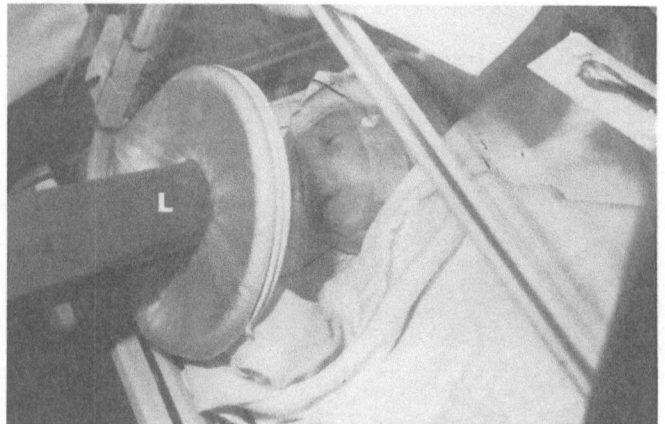

FIGURE 4-16.
Electroretinograms can be obtained in the nursery. The timing light (L) is placed in front of the eye to be tested after the child has been wired.

FIGURE 4-17.
VECP is being performed in the nursery. Light emission diodes (LED) goggles are indispensible when performing these electrophysiological tests.

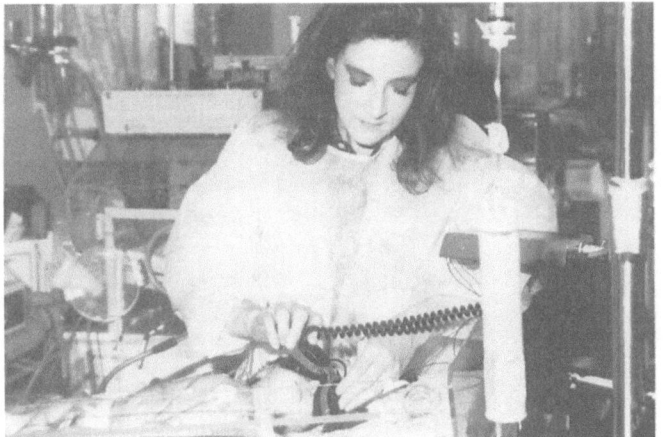

Section 2

Infectious Diseases

Chapter 5

Cysticercus

The larval form of the pork tapeworm *cysticercus cellulosae* remains an important cause of blindness in many parts of the world. The larvae grow within the small intestine of the human who has ingested contaminated pork. Usually heat destroys the organism, but if the pork is insufficiently cooked the larvae survive and grow into adults. The infested human then discharges ova in the feces, which are again ingested by swine.

Ocular structures seem to be a popular nesting ground for the ova, although they have also been seen in the aqueous, vitreous, and subretinal areas. Almost one half of patients with a cysticercus infection have ocular manifestations. Ultrasonographic evaluation of the vitreous cavity will demonstrate the cystic larva. Dead larvae are able to incite a massive inflammatory reaction in the eye. It generally affects young children and can be seen bilaterally. Surgical removal is the best form of therapy. Histopathological examination will demonstrate a scolex present in the specimen.

Suggested Reading

Hutton WL, Vaiser A, Snyder WB (1976). Pars plana vitrectomy for removal of intravitreous Cysticercus. Am J Ophthalmol 81:571-573

Zinn KM, Guillory SL, Friedman AH (1980). Removal of intravitreous cystercerci from the surface of the optic nerve head. Arch Ophthalmol 98:714-716

Figures

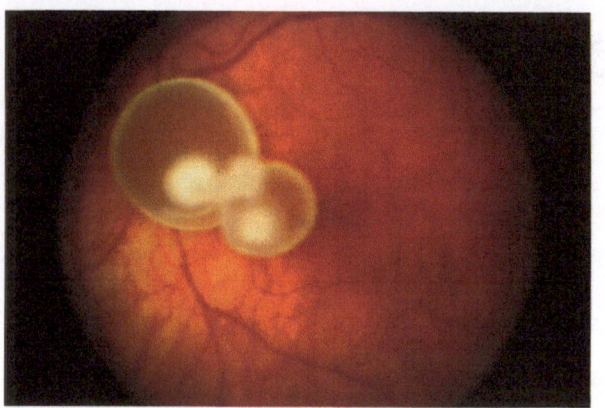

A

FIGURE 5-1.
(A) *Cysticercus* present in the vitreous cavity. It was removed via the standard three-port pars plana vitrectomy procedure. (From Zinn KM, Guillory SL, Friedman AH. Removal of intravitreous cysticerci from the surface of the optic nerve head. Arch Ophthalmol 98:714-716, 1980. With permission.) (B) The patient's acuity has been restored to a normal level. No complications were experienced by the patient.

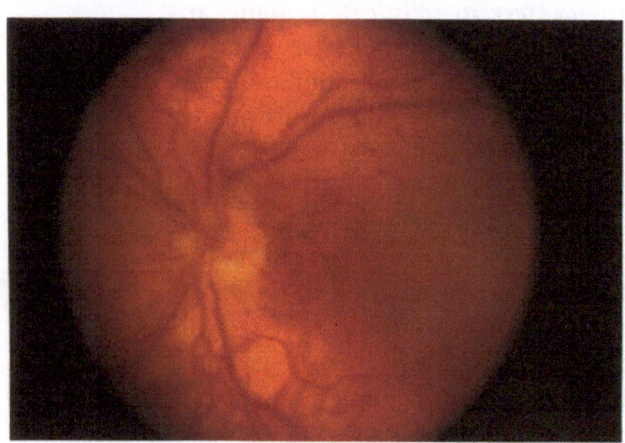

B

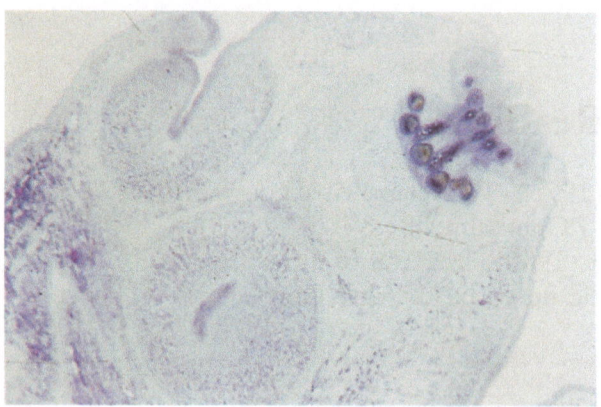

FIGURE 5-2.
On pathology examination the scolex is readily identified. (Toluidine blue)

FIGURE 5-3.
A *cysticercus* is present in the subretinal space. Careful examination reveals the scolex at the macula.

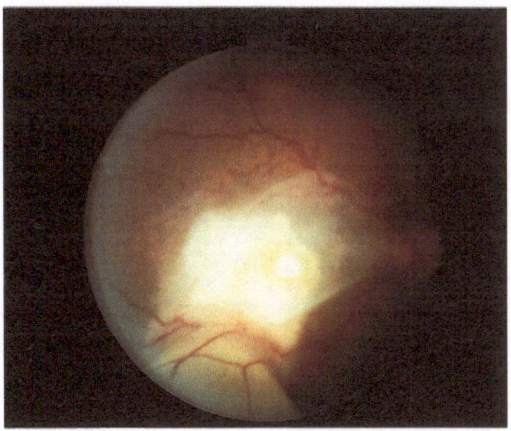

Chapter 6

Cytomegalic Inclusion Disease

Cytomegalovirus (CMV) is a ubiquitous DNA virus that is kept in check by our immune system. It is a member of the herpes family. Congenital infection is thought to result from maternal infection across the placenta or as the fetus passes through the birth canal. The infant usually has retinitis or choroiditis. The retinitis is a progressive one with extensive necrosis and hemorrhage. The vitritis that accompanies this disease is moderate, often mild in view of the extensive amount of retinal destruction.

Systemically, other organ systems may be affected in these children. Often there is hepatosplenomegaly concurrent with anemia, thrombocytopenia, and jaundice. Neurological problems may also be present. The features of congenital CMV disease may mimic those of congenital toxoplasmosis, especially when the infection is mild. With the advent of AIDS, CMV retinitis has become widespread. Up to 30% of AIDS patients with CMV retinitis can develop retinal detachments.

Histologically, a necrotizing retinitis is present. Cells show eosinophilic intranuclear inclusions and basophilic intracytoplasmic inclusions. The intracytoplasmic inclusions are the virions.

Selected Reading

Burns RP (1959). Cytomegalic inclusion disease uveitis: report of a case with isolation from aqueous humor of the virus in tissue culture. Arch Ophthalmol 61:376-387

Friedman AH, Orellana J, Freeman WR (1983). Cytomeglovirus retinitis: A manifestation of the acquired immune deficiency syndrome (AIDS). Br J Ophthal 67:372-80

Orellana J, Teich SA, Lieberwan RM, Restrepo S, Peairs R (1991). Treatment of retinal detachment in patients with the acquired immune deficiency syndrome. Ophthalmology 98:939-943

Smith ME, Zimmerman LE, Harley RD (1966). Ocular involvement in congenital cytomegalic inclusion disease. Arch Ophthalmol 76:696-699

Figures

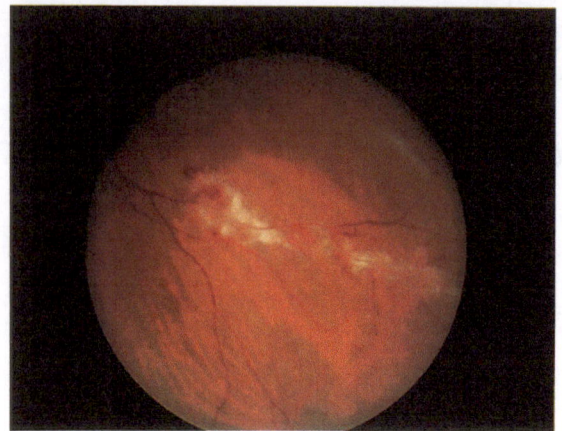

FIGURE 6-1.
Congenital cytomegalic inclusion disease can be unilateral and is usually seen in the posterior fundus. This person has perivascular involvement with hemorrhage and necrosis of the retina. There is minimal overlying vitreous reaction.

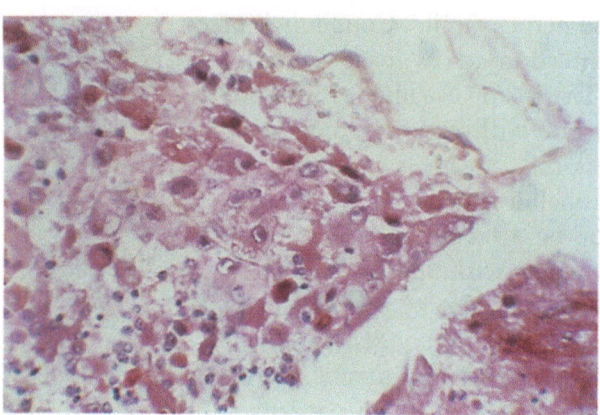

FIGURE 6-2.
Histopathology demonstrates retinal necrosis. The large cells contain basophilic intranuclear and intracytoplasmic inclusions. (H & E)

Chapter 7

Herpes Simplex

Herpes simplex retinitis in the newborn is usually due to type II infection contracted from the maternal genital tract. In addition to the necrotizing retinitis, there can also be focal white infiltrates as well as heaping of the retinal pigment epithelium (RPE). Neurological disturbances are always present as a sequelae of the infection. The child may have a co-existing encephalitis. Treatment of these children is with intravenous acyclovir, which may help the associated skin lesions resolve. In young adults, keratitis, iridocyclitis or chorioretinitis can be seen. Treatment for the keratitis can be lengthy while the uveitic manifestations can be difficult to control.

Histologically, there is retinal necrosis with reaction of the RPE. The RPE forms a hyperplastic plaque where the necrosis is present.

Selected Reading

Cogan DG, Kuwabara T, Young GF, et al (1964). Herpes simplex retinopathy in an infant. Arch Ophthalmol 72:641-645

Cibis GW (1975). Neonatal herpes simplex retinitis. Graefes Arch Klin Exp Ophthalmol 196:39-47

Figures

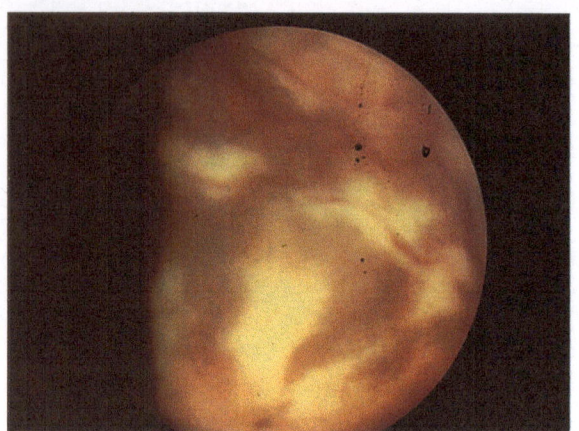

FIGURE 7-1.
Herpes simplex retinitis often appears as extensive yellow-white infiltrates and retinal hemorrhages. The disease is usually associated with type II virus.

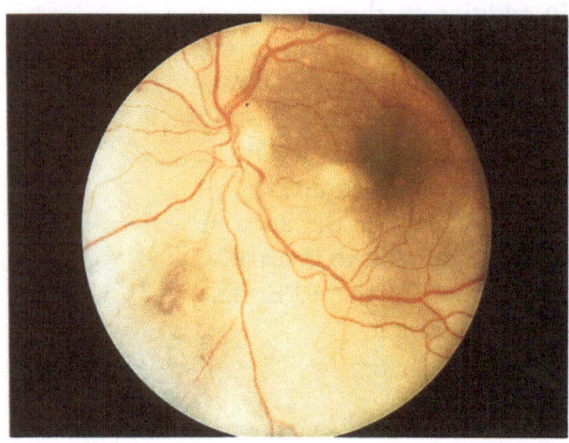

FIGURE 7-2.
This patient had herpes simplex retinitis encephalitis. Most cases are associated with central nervous system involvement.

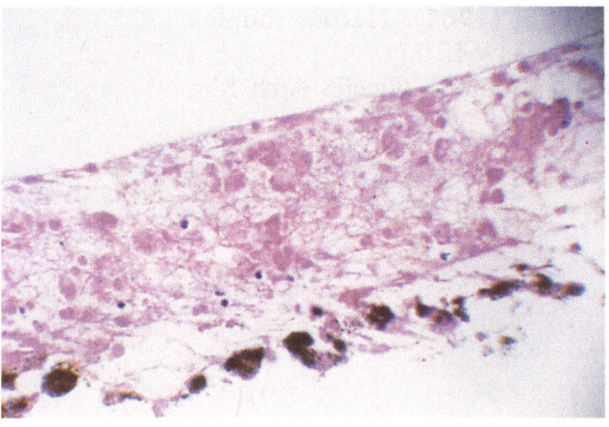

FIGURE 7-3.
Histopathology demonstrates retinal necrosis and chronic inflammatory cell infiltration. (H & E)

FIGURE 7-4.
Herpes simplex virus (HSV) as revealed by
peroxidase stain.

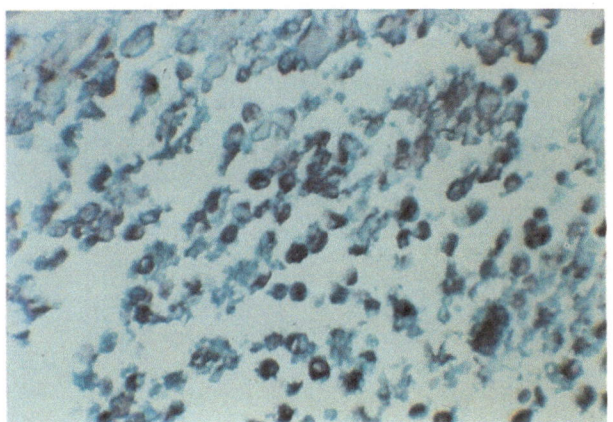

FIGURE 7-4.

Chapter 8

Luetic Chorioretinitis

Congenital syphilis usually presents with a constellation of systemic and ocular findings. Ocular manifestations include cataracts, glaucoma, and, during the second decade of life, interstitial keratitis. Optic atrophy, vessel attenuation, and a peripheral "salt and pepper" fundus are the usual keys to this diagnosis. The fundal picture is often mistaken for retinitis pigmentosa. Systemic findings include Hutchinson's teeth (pointed incisors), a broad saddle nose, bowed tibias, osteochondritis, and hepatosplenomegaly.

Visual acuity is normal unless interstitial keratitis is present. Visual fields, color vision, and electrophysiology are normal. The fluorescein angiogram depicts choroidal or pigment epithelial abnormalities.

Histologically, congenital lues is associated with nongranulomatous interstitial keratitis or anterior uveitis. In cases where there is posterior uveitis (acquired lues), atrophic retinal scars are surrounded by hyperplastic pigment epithelium. Congenital syphilis must be treated, usually with penicillin.

Selected Reading

Belin MW, Baltch AL, Hay PB (1981). Secondary syphilitic uveitis. Am J Ophthalmol 92:210-214

Friberg TR (1989). Syphilitic chorioretinitis. Arch Ophthalmol 107:1676-1677

Ryan SJ, Hardy PH, Hardy JM, et al (1972). Persistence of virulent Treponema pallidum despite penicillin therapy in congenital syphilis. Am J Ophthalmol 73:258-261

Figures

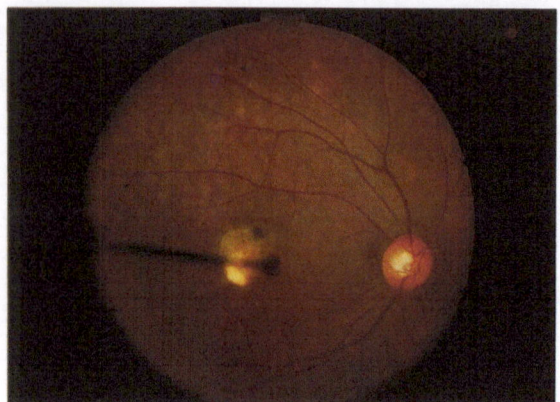

FIGURE 8-1.
Typical salt and pepper fundus of a patient with congenital lues. The patient also had a subretinal neovascular membrane.

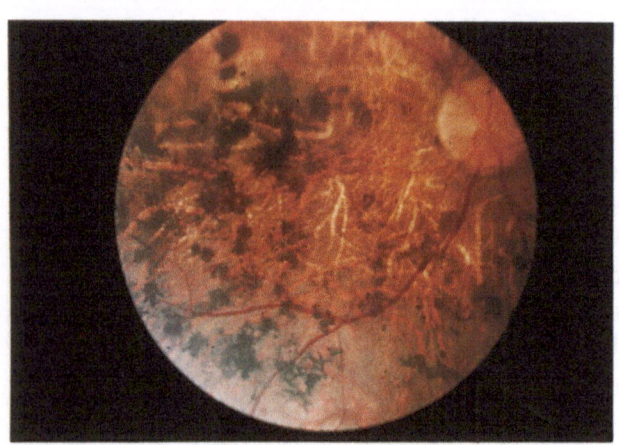

FIGURE 8-2.
Widespread chorioretinal atrophy with hyperplasia of the pigment epithelium.

FIGURE 8-3.
(A) Multiple chorioretinal scars are present, as well as some temporal optic atrophy. (B) This calotte shows the multiple lesions present in the fundus. (C) Areas of choroidal invasion by RPE cells are evident. This sign is considered pathognomonic by some ocular pathologists. (H & E)

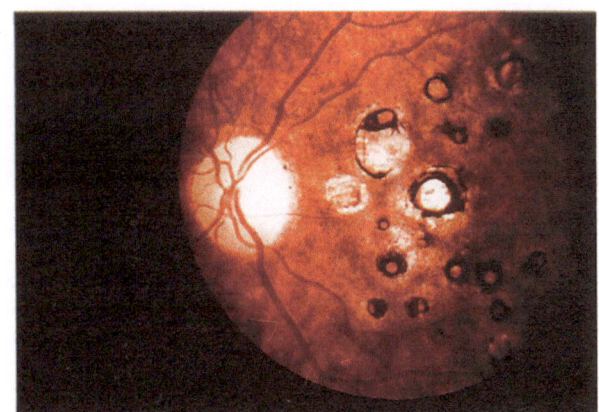

A

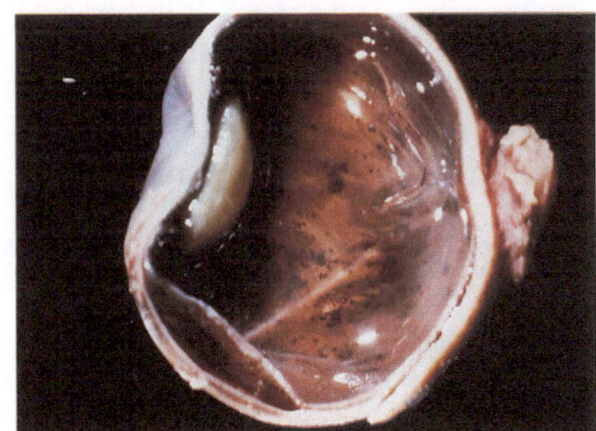

B

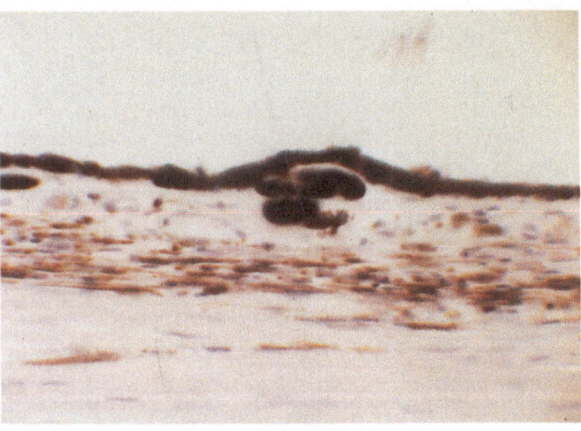

C

Chapter 9

Rubella Retinopathy

The differential diagnosis of a "salt and pepper" fundus includes rubella retinopathy. Because most children with rubella have a constellation of other signs, it is easy to determine the diagnosis. These patients have deafness and cataracts that are present at birth or develop postnatally. The lenses show persistent nucleated epithelial cells in the cortex. Other ocular signs are glaucoma (due to incomplete angle cleavage) and microphthalmos. Systemically, these children may have abnormalities of the brain and heart. It is important that these lenses are removed carefully, as viruses are shed on extraction, which can produce an overwhelming uveitis. Phthisis bulbi may be the sequelae of an uneventful cataract procedure.

Electrophysiological testing reveals no abnormalities, which helps to differentiate this condition from retinitis pigmentosa. The electroretinogram (ERG) in rubella tends to be normal in those with rubella, whereas it is abnormal in retinitis pigmentosa patients. The fluorescein angiogram merely documents multiple hypofluorescent spots corresponding to the areas of pigment mottling that make up the "salt and pepper" fundus.

Histopathologically, the lens in these patients has retained lens nuclei in the embryonic lens nucleus. It is not unusual to observe anterior and posterior lens degenerative changes as well. The ciliary body demonstrates necrosis as well as a chronic granulomatous reaction. The clinical "salt and pepper" fundus results from the alternation of retinal pigment epithelial (RPE) atrophy and hypertrophy.

Selected Reading

Collis WJ, Cohen DN (1970). Rubella retinopathy: a progressive disorder. Arch Ophthalmol 84:33-35

Wolff SM (1972). The ocular manifestations of congenital rubella. Trans Am Ophthalmol Soc 70:577-580

Yanoff M, Schaffer DB, Scheie HG (1968). Rubella ocular syndrome: clinical significance of viral and pathologic studies. Trans Am Acad Ophthalmol Otolaryngol 72:89-92

Figures

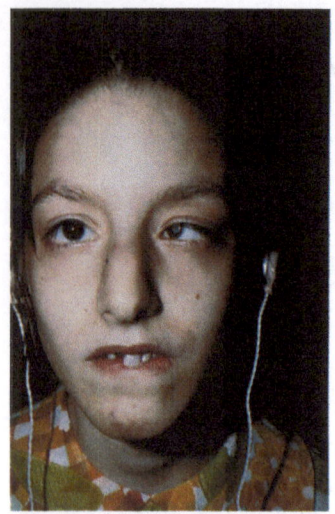

FIGURE 9-1.
Children with rubella typically have hearing problems as well as cataracts, cardiac problems, and mental retardation. This patient had congenital rubella and shows many signs of the disease.

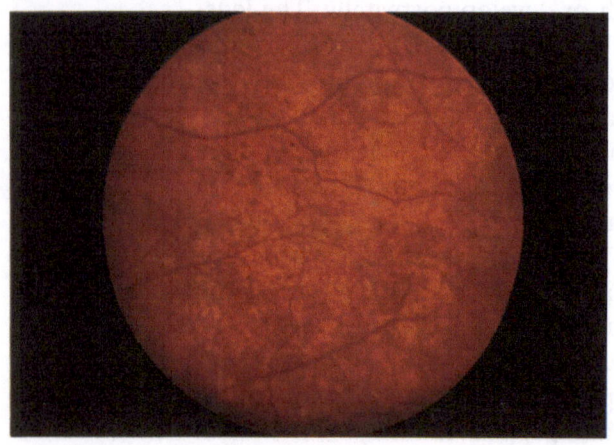

FIGURE 9-2.
Retina with pigment epithelial stippling. Atrophy and hypertrophy alternate giving the fundus a "salt and pepper" appearance.

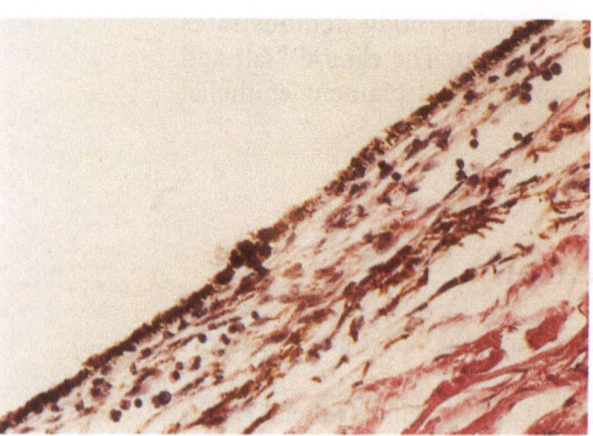

FIGURE 9-3.
Retinal pigment epithelial changes that produce the clinical picture. On the left there is RPE atrophy and on the right hypertrophy. (H & E)

Chapter 10

Toxocara Canis

The secondary larvae of the canine roundworm, *Toxocara canis*, attacks the liver, lungs, eyes, and brain. This condition, frequently called visceral larva migrans (VLM) syndrome, is an important cause of blindness in children. The ocular component of VLM is called ocular larval migrans, or OLM. It is frequently mistaken for retinoblastoma. The larva is absorbed into the system from the small intestine of children who have been infected while playing with puppies harboring the parasite. Because of its penetration into the central nervous system, these children may present with symptoms mimicking epilepsy or even a brain tumor. Ophthalmoscopically, a pseudoglioma may be present owing to the long standing presence of the larvae and the body's immunological reaction to it. The larva, which is minute, is rarely seen during the acute stages of the infection. When seen during late disease, it may be observed in the temporal quadrants. It is best noted using serial photography over many visits. There may be retinal edema with a small hemorrhage at the site where the larva is present. As time progresses, there is more and more exudation as well as host reaction, making it difficult to see the larva. Patients with the chronic infection demonstrate the characteristic granuloma in either the posterior pole or periphery. The granuloma represents multiple bouts of chorioretinitis over a long period.

Thiabendazole is the treatment of choice, although therapy must be given when the larva has not yet become encapsulated. Destruction of the larva *in situ* has been documented. In children who have acquired the larva and have a granuloma, pars plana removal of the granuloma has been successful. In some cases the child develops an endophthalmitis. Electophysiological evaluation of these particular cases is important. The retinal destruction that may take place must be evaluated before surgery is contemplated.

Selected Reading

Ashton N (1960). Larval granulomatosis of the retina due to Toxocara. Br J Ophthalmol 44:129-148

Nichols RL (1956). The etiology of visceral larva migrans: diagnostic morphology of infective second-stage Toxocara larvae. J Parasitol 42:349-362

Siam AL (1973). Toxocaral chorioretinitis: treatment of early cases with photocoagulation. Br J Ophthalmol 57:700-703

Wan WL, Cano MR, Pince KJ, Green RL (1991). Echographic characteristics of ocular toxocariasis. Ophthalmology 98:28-32

Wilder HC (1950). Nematode endophthalmitis. Trans Am Acad Ophthalmol Otolaryngol 55:99-109

Figures

FIGURE 10-1.
This pateint with toxocariasis has a clear media and a discrete lesion in the macula.

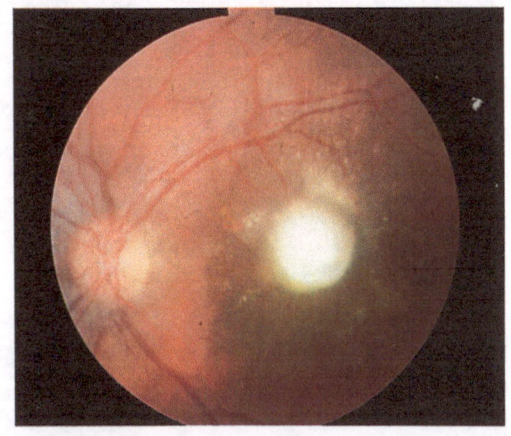

FIGURE 10-2.
This child was referred from Trinidad for evaluation of the right eye. The patient had toxocariasis, and a peripheral white lesion is easily visible. There were some retinal folds.

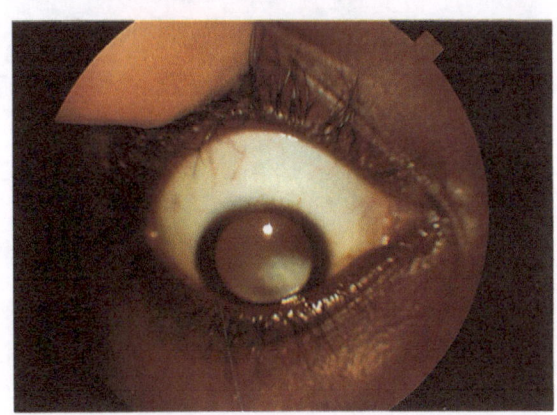

FIGURE 10-3.
Retina had been detached. Demarcation lines are easily visible in the areas not containing the granuloma. An electroretinogram (ERG) did not demonstrate a recordable a- or b-wave. Surgery was not offered to the patient. The ERG in the fellow, uninvolved eye was normal.

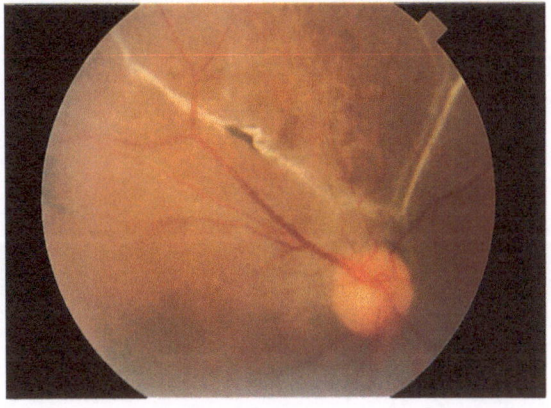

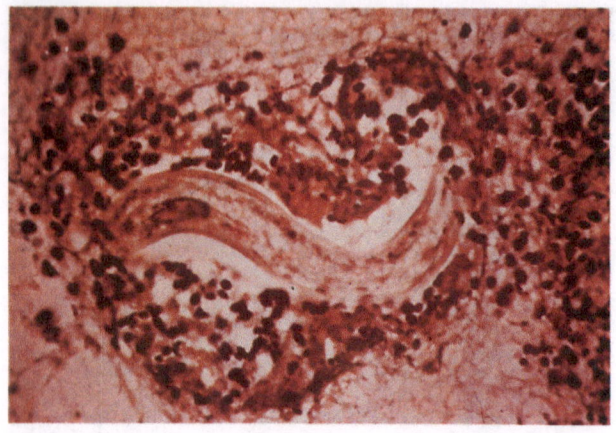

FIGURE 10-4.
On occasion, so much granulomatous inflammation is present there is leukocoria. Pars plana vitrectomy with removal of the necrotic worm is possible. This specimen demonstrates the worm surrounded by many inflammatory cells. (H & E)

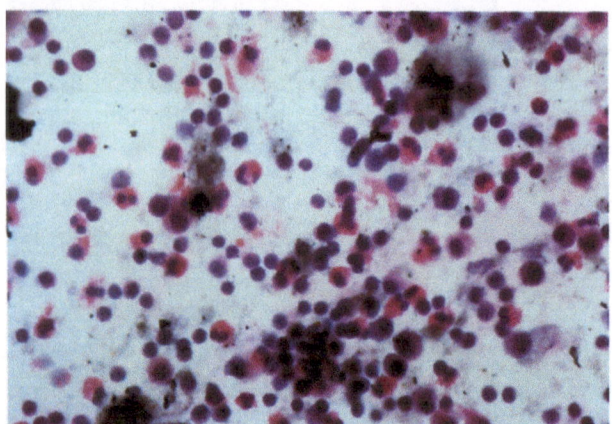

FIGURE 10-5.
Careful analysis of these inflammatory cells demonstrates that they are eosinophils (pink cytoplasm) and neutrophils. (H & E)

Chapter 11

Toxoplasmosis

Serological evidence that children have toxoplasmosis may be present without evidence of clinical disease. Toxoplasmosis is caused by toxoplasma gondii which is an obligate intracellular parasite. The fetuses acquire the disease from the mother who becomes infected while pregnant. The classic signs of congenital toxoplasmosis include fever, jaundice, chorioretinitis, intracranial calcifications on radiographic studies, hydrocephalus, and convulsions. Infants may be born with the disease, or it may not become apparent until the infant is almost 1 year old. The immunoglobulin M (IgM) fluorescent antibody test is diagnostic for the disease.

The disease begins as a coagulative necrosis of the retina that spreads into the vitreous. The underlying choroid may show a granulomatous reaction sometimes involving the sclera. In the vitreous there is marked inflammation over each of the foci of infection. Most cases of congenital toxoplasmosis consist of one lesion—a macular lesion in 40% of cases. The lesions can be multifocal and can be seen bilaterally. With time, the lesions heal with the characteristic hyperpigmented ring. In those cases where there are frequent reactivations, xenon arc photocoagulation of the lesion and surrounding retina may be of benefit in preventing further reactivation. The vitritis may become so severe that retinal details are obscured.

Therapy of toxoplasmosis has been a subject of some controversy. Standard therapy includes clindamycin, sulfonamide, and pyrimethamine with folinic acid. Some authors add oral prednisone. Most recently a drug, called 566C80 (Burroughs Welcome), has been used to successfully treat toxoplasmosis.

Selected Reading

Desmonts G, Couvreur J, Ben Rachid MS (1965). Le toxoplasme, la mere et l'enfant. Arch Fr Pediatr 22:1183-1200

Francois J (1963). Traitement de la toxoplasmose (etude experimintale). Bull Soc Belge Ophtalmol 134:354-361

Lopez JS, de Smet MC, Masur H, et al (1992). Orally administered 566C80 for treatment of ocular toxoplasmosis in a patient with the acquired immunodeficiency syndrome. Am J Ophthalmol 113:331-333

Remington JS (1969). The present status of the IgM fluorescent antibody technique in the diagnosis of congenital toxoplasmosis. J Pediatr 75:1116-1124

Figures

FIGURE 11-1.
Congenital toxoplasmosis is associated with encephalomyelitis, visceral disease, and retinochoroiditis. Typically, as in this case, there is a large chorioretinal scar at the macula. The disease reactivates various times throughout the patient's life. Because of the position of the lesion, this person's acuity is at the level of hand motion.

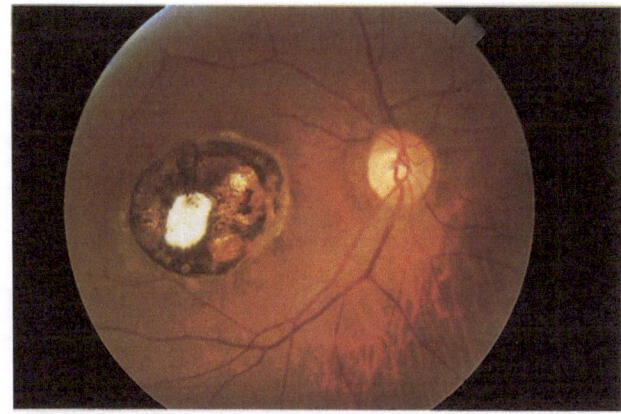

FIGURE 11-2.
Fortunately for this patient, the toxoplasmosis lesion is located away from the posterior pole. The lesion is active, producing a vitritis. On occasion, the vitritis is so severe the retina cannot be visualized. Macular edema may develop.

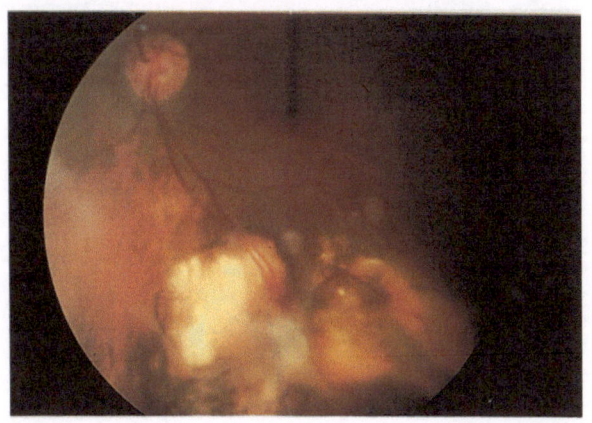

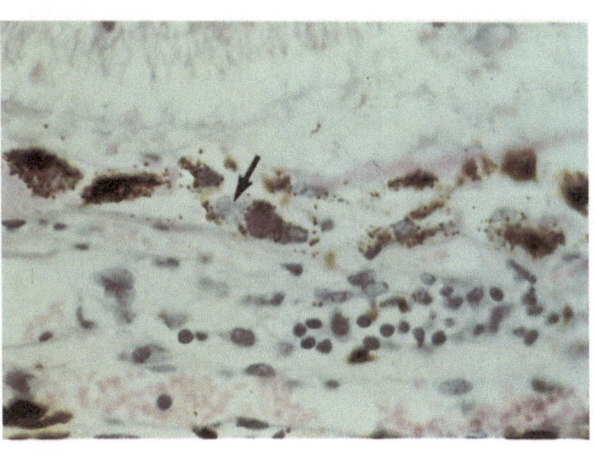

FIGURE 11-3.
Histopathology demonstrates a cyst (arrow) in a retinal pigment epithelial cell.

Section 3

Vitreoretinal Degenerations

Chapter 12

Goldmann-Favre Syndrome

Goldmann-Favre syndrome, also known as recessive hyaloideoretinal dystrophy, is one of the inherited vitreoretinal degenerative disorders. Inherited by the autosomal recessive modes, it is the only vitreoretinal degeneration inherited in such a fashion; the other forms of vitreoretinal degeneration are autosomal dominant and in one case X-linked. Although the condition is not seen frequently, it shares many aspects with X-linked retinoschisis (another vitreoretinal degeneration). The sexes are affected equally. Goldmann-Favre syndrome patients complain of night blindness (usually during the first decade of life) and typically have significant myopia and progressive constriction of their visual fields. As with X-linked retinoschisis, there is both macular and peripheral schisis with pigmentary alterations (bone corpuscle type) and chorioretinal atrophy. The cystoid-appearing macula can take on a beaten-copper appearance. The vitreous undergoes liquefaction with the presence of fibrous strands of varying thickness. Preretinal membranes can also be seen.

Fluorescein angiography demonstrates large areas of peripheral nonperfusion. Fluorescein leakage from capillaries at the macula, periphery, and edges of the schisis cavities can be seen. As the disease progresses, cataracts may be present. The Farnsworth-Munsell 100 hue test brings out blue-yellow defects, and the pseudoisochromatic plates show a red-green deficiency. Electroretinographic findings show a minimal response, and the pattern is often extinct. The electrooculogram may also be abnormal. Ultimately, there is a profound loss of acuity. Retinal detachment tends to be technically difficult to repair and frequently prophylactic therapy is advocated for tears even in patients one would otherwise not treat.

Selected Reading

Favre M (1958). A propos de deux cas de degenerescence hyaloideore-tinienne. Ophthalmologica 135:604-609

Fishman GA, Jampol LM, Goldberg MF (1976). Diagnostic features of Favre-Goldmann syndrome. Br J Ophthalmol 60:345-353

Goldmann H (1957). Biomicroscopie de corps vitre et du fond de l'oeil. Bull Mem Soc Fr Ophthalmol 70:265

Figures

FIGURE 12-1.
Young woman with nyctalopia. Note the schisis inferiorly with multiple vitreous membranes. Over the years, the schisis cavity has flattened.

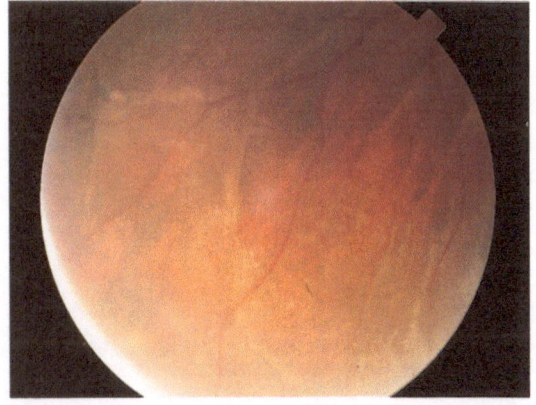

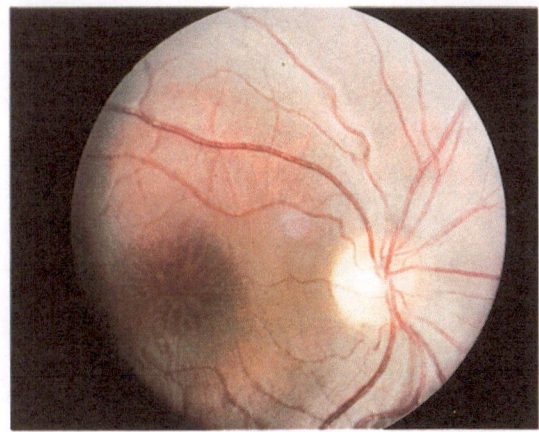

FIGURE 12-2.
Macula shows cystoid degeneraton. The disc is normal.

Chapter 13

Familial Exudative Vitreoretinopathy

Criswick and Schepens coined the name familial exudative vitreoretinopathy (FEVR) in 1969. The condition appears to have various ways of expressing itself. Usually the eye demonstrates temporal dragging of the retina, producing a loss of acuity over several weeks. Many cases have subretinal exudates, and a fluorescein angiogram can document the extensive peripheral nonperfusion present in almost 90% of the eyes. Other retinal signs are detachments, peripheral cystoid degeneration, neovascularization, and vitreous bands. FEVR is inherited in an autosomal dominant fashion with a high degree of penetrance. There are many mild forms, and an individual may have a mild form in one eye and a severe form in the fellow eye. Retinopathy of prematurity (ROP) should be ruled out before FEVR is considered. Often the severe form of FEVR resembles Stage V ROP. More than 80% of patients have myopia. Color vision and electrophysiological testing tends to be normal. The entire family should be examined when a child presents with a picture of FEVR. Treatment is aimed towards the specific problems, such as photocoagulation or cryopexy of neovascular lesions. Histopathology demonstrates neovascularization (retinal and iris) fibrovascular membranes and exudates.

Selected Reading

Criswick VG, Schepens CL (1969). Familial exudative vitreoretinopathy. Am J Ophthalmol 68:578-594

Ober RR, Bird AC, Hamilton AM, et al (1980). Autosomal dominant exudative vitreoretinopathy. Br J Ophthalmol 64:112-120

Figures

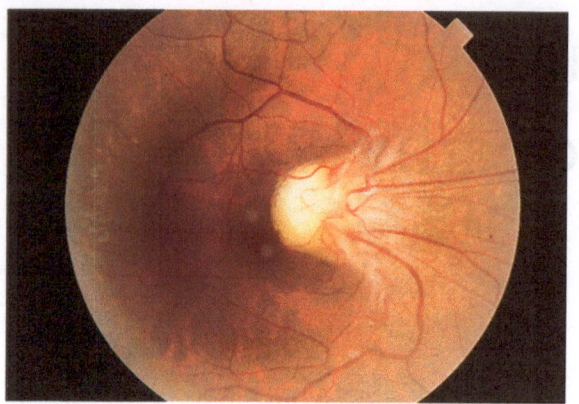

A

FIGURE 13-1.
(A) Pseudoexotropia in the right eye. Note the extreme temporal dragging of the retina. The macula was in a falciform fold, and acuity was at the level of hand motions. (B) The fellow eye did not have the temporal dragging but did have peripheral membranes with peripheral cystoid changes.

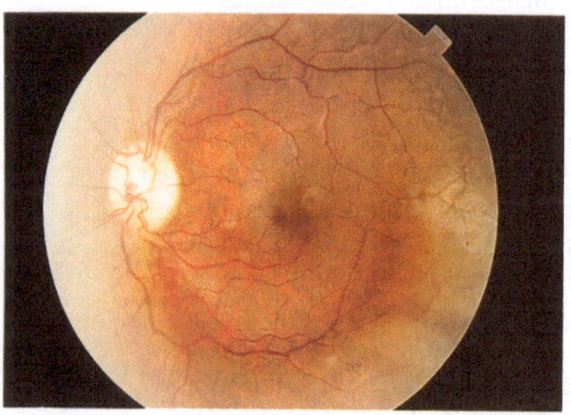

B

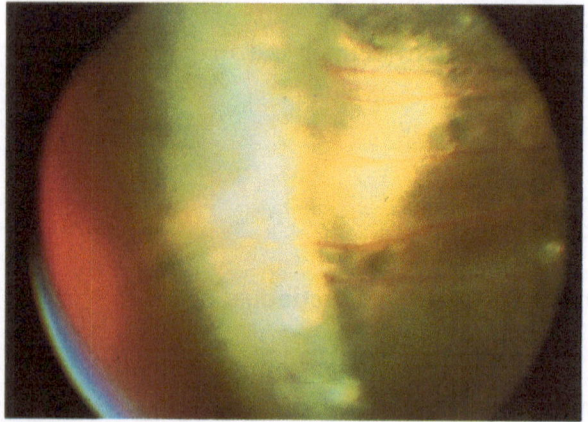

FIGURE 13-2.
Fibrovascular proliferative changes in the periphery of a patient with FEVR. The peripheral exudation can be readily seen.

FIGURE 13-3.
Fluorescein angiography demonstrates vascular changes. Note the vascular straightening and leakage.

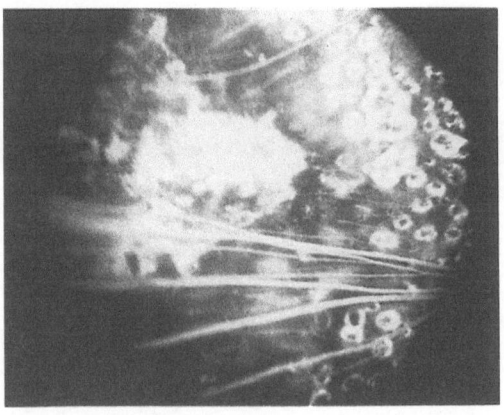

Chapter 14

Wagner Syndrome and Stickler Syndrome

The characteristic features of Wagner syndrome include myopia, an optically empty vitreous, preretinal membranes, perivascular retinal pigment epithelial changes, vascular sheathing, cataracts, and atrophy of the choriocapillaris. The cataracts typically appear as patients approach their 40th birthday. The vitreous bands are broad and insert into the peripheral retina; and there is liquefaction of the vitreous. It is autosomal dominant and usually present bilaturally. It is noteworthy that many physicians consider Wagner syndrome to be a mild form of Stickler syndrome. Wagner syndrome patients, however, do not have systemic changes, whereas Stickler syndrome patients have systemic manifestations. The former patients do not suffer retinal detachments, whereas more than 50% of the Stickler syndrome patients develop a retinal detachment.

Visual acuity is normal if both the posterior pole and lens are normal. Color vision is usually normal. Although the electroretinogram is normal early in the disease, as time progresses it becomes more and more abnormal.

The addition of systemic manifestations to Wagner syndrome encompasses the entity known as Stickler syndrome, or hereditary progressive arthroophthalmopathy. As with Wagner syndrome, it is a progressive hereditary disorder with an autosomal dominant pattern of inheritance. The systemic aspects of this disease involve the facial and skeletal systems. The ocular signs of the disease are similar to those seen with Wagner syndrome. The myopia (usually more than 10 diopters), retinal breaks, cataracts, and glaucoma appear to be progressive in this disorder. The prognosis for retinal detachment surgery is usually unfavorable. It is estimated that at least 50% of these patients experience a detachment during their lifetime. These patients also seem to have a high incidence of hearing loss. They have flattened facies, a cleft palate, and arthropathy. Stickler syndrome patients can be categorized into four subgroups, as was done by Lisch in 1983: (1) those with facial abnormalities and a cleft palate; (2) those with an Eskimo-like face; (3) those with hyperextensibility of joints and a cleft palate; and (4) those with progressive arthroophthalmopathy.

Color vision is unaffected in these patients. The visual fields may demonstrate constriction. Electrophysiological studies in Stickler syndrome patients are similar to those seen in patients with Wagner syndrome, that is, subnormal. Dark adaptation may be normal or abnormal. It should be remembered that retinal detachments and an oral cavity abnormality bespeaks of a variant of Stickler syndrome commonly known as "clefting syndromes."

Selected Reading

Alexander RL, Shea M (1965). Wagner's disease. Arch Ophthalmol 74:310-318

Lisch W (1983). Hereditary vitreoretinal degenerations. Dev Ophthalmol 8:1-90

Maumenee IH (1979). Vitreoretinal degeneration as a sign of generalized connective tissue diseasses. Am J Ophthalmol 88:432-449

Maumenee IH, Stoll HU, Mets MB (1982). The Wagner syndrome versus hereditary arthroophthalmopathy. Trans Am Ophthalmol Soc 80:349-365

Pinkers A, Jansen LMAA (1974). Wagner's syndrome (degeneratio-hyaloideo-retinalis hereditaria). Doc Ophthalmol 37:245-259

Stickler GB, Belau PG, Farrell FJ, et al (1965). Hereditary progressive arthro-ophthalmopathy. Mayo Clin Proc 40:433-455

Figures

FIGURE 14-1.
In this patient with Wagner syndrome, pigment has accumulated in the retina and choroid. Note also closure of a retinal vessel, which has become white.

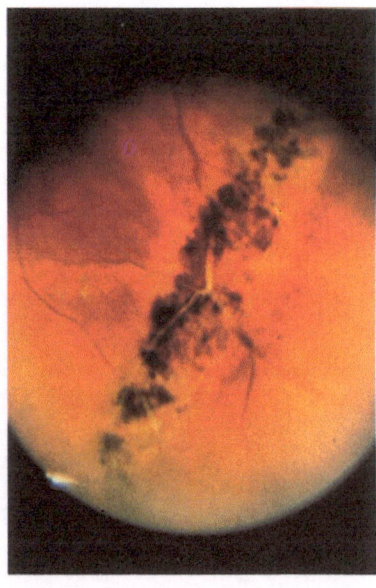

FIGURE 14-2.
Translucent, fenestrated membrane in a patient with Wagner syndrome.

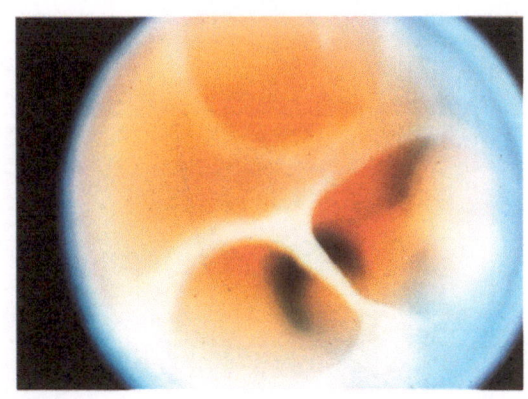

FIGURE 14-3.
This patient with Stickler syndrome had a flattened frontal bone and an underdeveloped mandible. A roentgenogram revealed a supernumerary carpal bone and shortened regular carpal bones. The patient had a sensorineural hearing loss as well. The fundus has equatorial membranes with peripheral retinal and choroidal pigmentation.

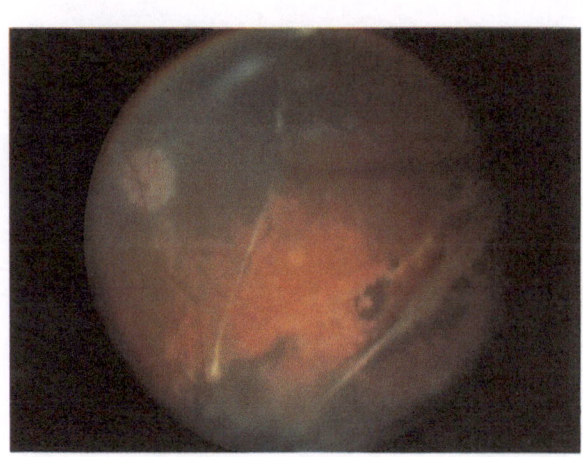

Chapter 15

Juvenile Retinoschisis

Juvenile retinoschisis often goes by other names, such as congenital schisis or, more commonly, X-linked retinoschisis. The condition is most commonly noted within the first year of life, and the presenting problem is that the child has noted decreased central acuity. Because the gene for this anomaly is present on the X chromosome, daughters are carriers and 50% of their male siblings have the disease.

Essentially, the disease involves the retina splitting into two parts. The split occurs in the nerve fiber layer, producing a bullous but tense elevation of the inner retina. This split is in contrast to the classic adult type of retinoschisis, where the split occurs in the outer plexiform layer. Inner breaks are not unusual, and on many occasions the holes are so large no tissue can be seen except for the blood vessels, which seem to be suspended. Additionally, there is one feature peculiar to juvenile retinoschisis: Nearly 100% of children with the disease have a stellate cystoid macula that demonstrates schisis. Vitreous hemorrhage from ruptured blood vessels or new vessels and optic atrophy may also be seen.

Complications from juvenile retinoschisis may occur. Retinal detachments are seen in about 20% of the patients. The vitreous veils seen in these eyes can be derived from the thin inner layers of the schisis.

Diagnostically, the fluorescein angiogram demonstrates window defects in the fovea that correspond to the schisis. The schisis does not leak fluorescein. Electrophysiological studies show a decreased scotopic b-wave, and the electrooculogram is normal. Oscillatory potentials are also decreased. Senile retinoschisis produces an electroretinogram with decreased a- and b-waves. Central scotomas are elicited by the central schisis, and absolute peripheral scotomas are caused by the peripheral schisis.

Therapy for this condition has been less than optimal. Because the complications of progressive splitting, extensive foveal schisis, retinal detachments, and vitreous hemorrhage may occur, therapy is aimed at each individual entity. A scleral buckle can be used to treat a retinal detachment, and vitreous hemorrhage may necessitate vitrectomy. Progressive foveal changes, however, cannot be stopped.

Selected Reading

Bloome MA, Garcia CA (1982). Manual of Retinal and Choroidal Dystrophies. Norwalk, CT: Appleton-Century-Crofts, pp. 25-29

Condon GP, Brownstein S, Wang NS, et al (1986). Congenital hereditary (juvenile X-linked) retinoschisis: histopathologic and ultrastructural findings in three eyes. Arch Ophthalmol 104:576-583

Tasman W (1975). Macular changes in congenital retinoschisis. Mod Probl Ophthalmol 15:40-49

Yanoff M, Rahn EK, Zimmerman LE (1968). Histopathology of juvenile retinoschisis. Arch Ophthalmol 79:49-53

Figures

FIGURE 15-1.
Foveal schisis is seen in almost 100% of cases of juvenile retinoschisis. This boy was 10 years old and had a brother age 7 who also had retinoschisis.

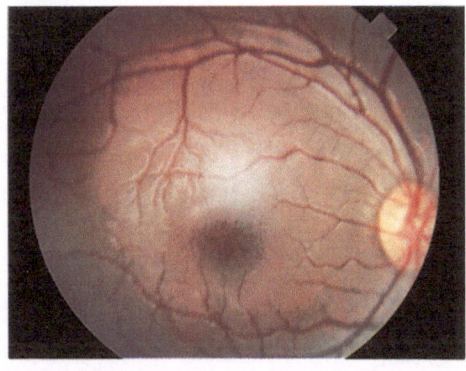

FIGURE 15-2.
Peripheral retinoschisis is present more than 50% of the time. The split is seen within the nerve fiber layer.

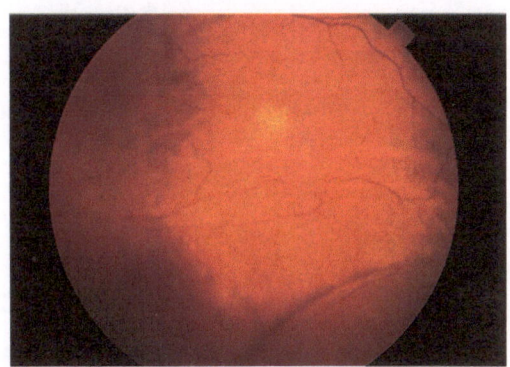

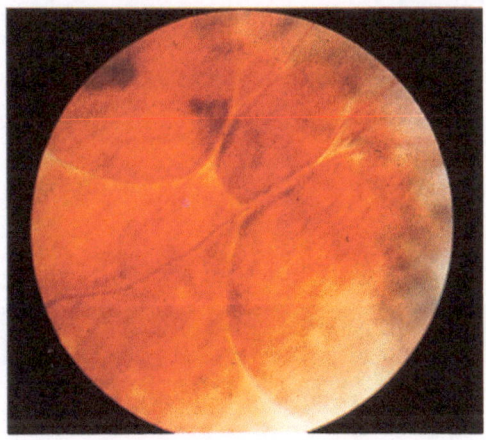

FIGURE 15-3.
The vessels are thin wires that appear to be suspended in the inner layers. Peripheral schisis can progress, as can macular schisis.

Section 4

Vascular Diseases

Chapter 16

Coats' Disease

Classically, patients with Coats' disease present with a leukocoria, strabismus, and poor vision. These patients are mostly male (3:1) and usually between 2 and 16 years of age. Certainly more than 66% of the cases appear before the end of the first decade of life. Some believe that there are patients who have presented at birth with Coats' disease.

More than half of the patients have strabismus, and about three-fourths of the cases are unilateral. Because of the retinal vascular abnormalities, massive exudative detachments are present. In extreme cases, neovascular glaucoma may be a problem.

Therapy is aimed at the abnormal telangiectatic vessels, which leak massively. Therapy is either photocoagulation or cryoretinopexy. Xenon arc photocoagulation is particularly effective in these children for preventing the development of a massive exudative response. Such responses can cause cataracts, glaucoma, and even phthisis of the eye.

Clinically, the picture is one of retinal elevation due to massive amounts of yellow subretinal exudate. Early in the disease, one sees quadrantic telangiectasia with intraretinal exudation. The vasculature in the area of exudation is often tortuous, with aneurysmal dilatations and sheathing. Hemorrhages are often seen. Later in the disease there is massive subretinal exudation.

Fluorescein angiography demonstrates the vascular abnormalities seen with this entity. Telangiectasia and aneurysmal dilatation are commonly seen on the angiogram. There is early leakage that persists throughout the angiogram. There may be areas of extensive capillary nonperfusion. Electrophysiology may become abnormal as the retinal detachment progresses. The disease usually progresses, but spontaneous resolution has been reported. Histopathology demonstrates irregular dilation of the vascular system with the PAS positive fluid in the outer retinal layers. Lipid laden macrophages can also be seen.

Selected Reading

Coats G (1908). Forms of retinal disease with massive exudation. R Lond Ophthalmol Hosp Rev 18:440-525

Deutsch TA, Rabb MF, Jampol LM (1982). Spontaneous regression of retinal lesions in Coats' disease. Can J Ophthalmol 17:169-172

Egerer I, Tasman W, Tomer TT (1974). Coats' disease. Arch Ophthalmol 92:109-112

Goel SD, Augsburger JJ (1991). Hemorrhagic retinal macrocysts in advanced Coats' disease. Retina 11:437-440

Harris G (1970). Coats' disease, diagnosis and treatment. Can J Ophthalmol 5:311-320

Ridley ME, Shields JA, Brown GC, Tasman WS (1982). Coats' disease, evaluation of management. Ophthalmology 89:1381-1387

Figures

FIGURE 16-1.
Exudative detachment of the retina with associated telangiectatic vessels, neovascularization, and saccular venous dilatation in a male teenager.

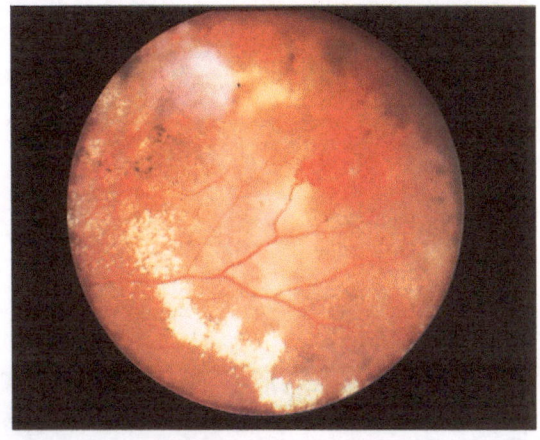

FIGURE 16-2.
Fluorescein angiogram clearly shows the exudation. The superior part suggests nonperfusion.

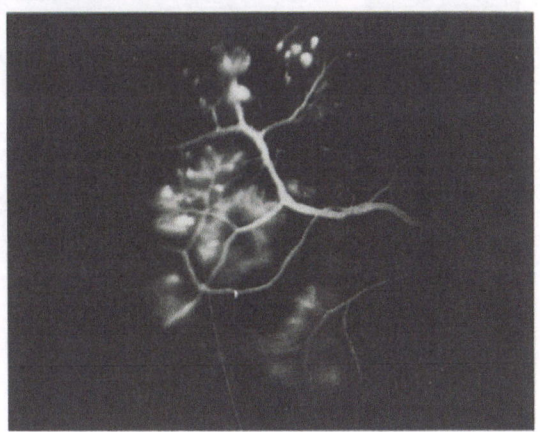

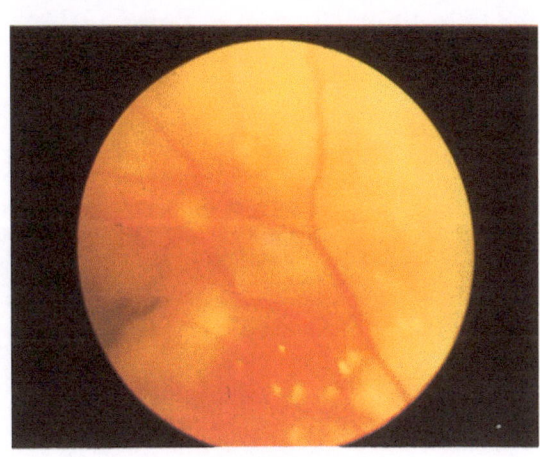

FIGURE 16-3.
Extensive exudation is present. As the exudation progresses, glaucoma may result.

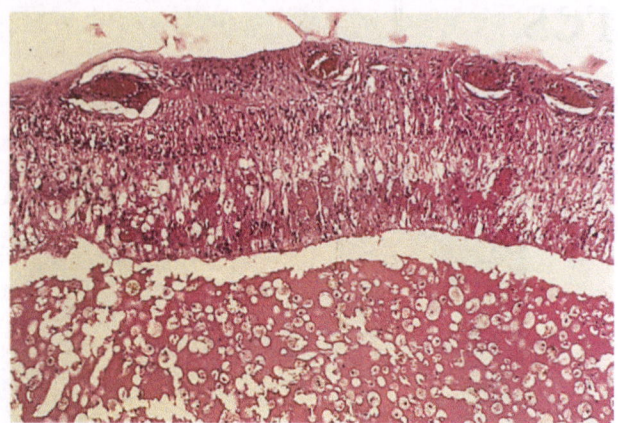

FIGURE 16-4.
Intraretinal exudation. Note the subretinal collection of foam-laden histiocytes. (H & E)

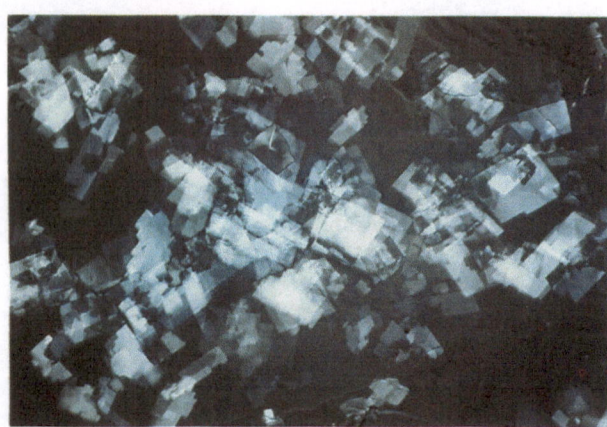

FIGURE 16-5.
Cholesterol crystals in the subretinal exudate. (Photomicrograph with polarized light)

Chapter 17

Eales' Disease

Idiopathic periphlebitis in men has come to be known as Eales' disease. Typically men (in their third decade) with this entity are affected bilaterally and often present with a vitreous hemorrhage. Periphlebitis is often followed by increasingly larger areas of capillary nonperfusion and ultimately neovascularization. Severe visual loss ensues when the complications of rubeosis, hemorrhage, and glaucoma become predominant.

The diagnosis of Eales' disease is made by exclusion. All other causes of peripheral neovascularization and periphlebitis must be ruled out. The most commonly associated sign is auditory abnormalities. There has been a continued suggestion that patients with Eales' disease have an associated hypersensitivity reaction/allergic abnormalities because almost all Eales' disease patients have a positive tuberculin skin test. There may be a loose connection with collagen vascular disorders, sarcoidosis, and multiple sclerosis. Therapy is directed towards obliterating the neovascular fronds which cause vitreous hemorrhages. In severe cases, vitrectomy with endophotocoagulation is necessary.

Selected Reading

Eales H (1882). Primary retinal hemorrhage in young men. Ophthalmol Rev 1:41-46

Elliot AJ (1975). Thirty-year observation of patients with Eales' disease. Am J Ophthalmol 80:404-408

Renie WA, Murphy RP, Anderson KC, et al (1983). The evaluation of patients with Eales' disease. Retina 3:243-248

Figures

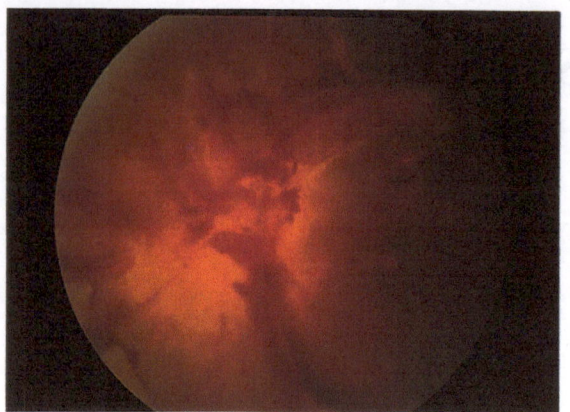

FIGURE 17-1.
A 25-year old man lost one eye to this vitreous hemorrhage and retinal detachment. He presented with periphlebitis and occlusive disease. He had a markedly positive PPD reaction with a weak antigen.

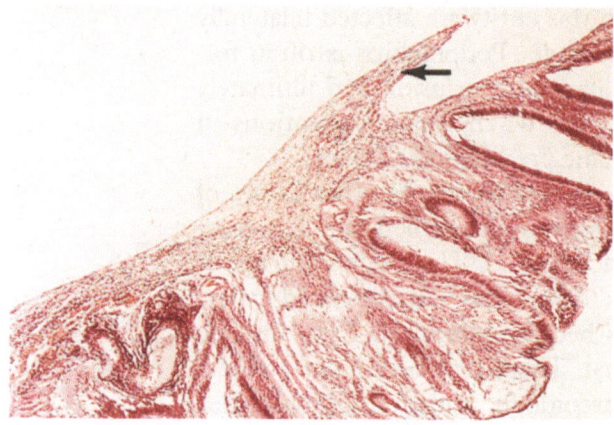

FIGURE 17-2.
This patient had multiple occlusive events in the posterior pole in this eye. Florid retinitis proliferans can be seen in the mid periphery. (H & E) (arrow)

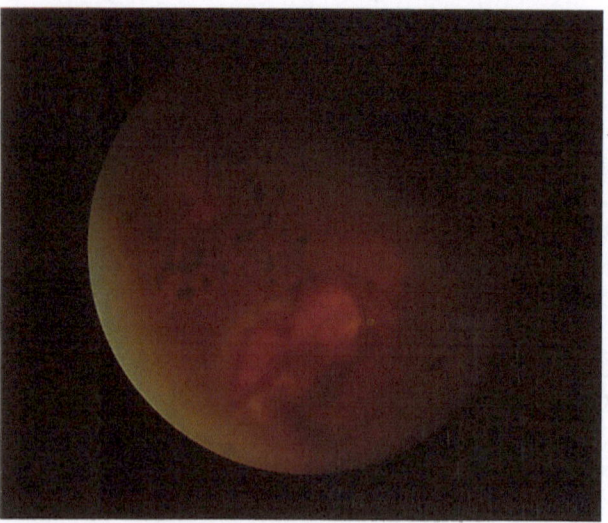

FIGURE 17-3.
Clinical photograph demonstrating peripheral neovascularization. Laser photocoagulation has been applied to one of these fronds.

FIGURE 17-4.
Fluorescein angiogram showing the hyperfluorescence seen in the peripheral neovascular fronds.

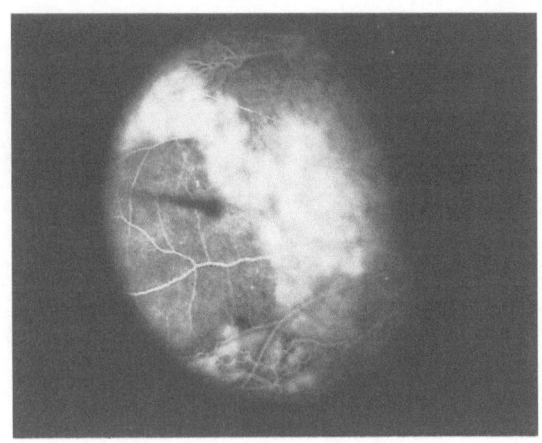

Chapter 18

Retinopathy of Prematurity

In 1942 Terry described several children who had leukocoria and a clear lens. He postulated that this entity represented an overgrowth of the vascular tunica. Since then we have learned that this retinopathy occurs to a great degree in premature children. A plethora of factors have been incriminated over time, such as oxygen, sepsis, shifting of the oxygen curve, and bronchodysplasia. These children seem to be born with a fair amount of undeveloped retina, as vascularization is not completed until 1 month after birth. It is a switch from orderly angiogenesis to disorderly proliferation that produces the retinopathy of prematurity (ROP).

A classification based on the extent and position of the abnormality has been established. The position of the disease is denoted by three zones.

Zone 1: Distance from the optic disc to twice the disc macular distance in all directions

Zone 2: from the outer border of zone 1 to the nasal ora and to the equator temporally

Zone 3: from the outer border of zone 2 to the remaining ora

The extent of the disease is expressed as the hours of a clock. Staging denotes the amount of disease present.

> Stage 1: demarcation line
> Stage 2: ridge formation
> Stage 3: ridge with extraretinal proliferation
> Stage 4A: subtotal detachment—uninvolved macula
> Stage 4B: subtotal detachment—involved macula
> Stage 5: total retinal detachment

Using this classification, communications among investigators and treatment results are easier to comprehend. Cryotherapy has been suggested by the Cryotherapy Study Group. The threshold indications are five or more contiguous clock hours or 8 cumulative clock hours of stage 3 disease in eye zone 1 or 2 with plus disease. In patients with a retinal detachment encroaching on the macula, a scleral buckle should be considered. Children with stage 5 disease, may benefit from closed vitrectomy or open sky vitrectomy.

After the active disease has abated, cicatricial disease becomes evident. The vascular system is pulled temporally, with temporal pigmentation appearing later. These patients have perivascular and radially oriented lattice lesions, peripheral schisis, and break formation.

Fluorescein angiography in ROP patients typically demonstrates vascular leakage due to the extensive neovascularization. The electroretinogram changes as the retina detaches, with loss of the a-wave and then the b-wave. Visual field defects are variable in cicatricial disease depending on how much retina has been distorted.

Histologically, it has been theorized that the spindle cells (vascular precursors) undergo transformation from a vasoformative role to that of vasoproliferation. It is manifested by an increase in gap junctions between these spindle cells. In stage I disease the demarcation line is set up by arteriovenous collaterals. Multiple microvascular abnormalities can be seen in this region. As retinitis proliferans develops, the vessels grow through the internal limiting membrane into the subvitreal space and eventually into the vitreous. Contracture of these vessels can cause the hemorrhages, and the fibrocellular components parallel to the shunt cause contraction and elevation of the shunt.

Selected Reading

Bradford JD (1991). Management of advanced retinopathy of prematurity in the older patient. Ophthalmology 98:1105-1109

Campbell K (1951). Intensive oxygen therapy as a possible cause of retrolental fibroplasia: a clinical approach. Med J Aust 2:48-50

Committee for the Classification of Retinopathy of Prematurity (1984). An international classification of retinopathy of prematurity. Arch Ophthalmol 102:1130-1134

Eichenbaum JW, Mamelok A, Mittl RN, Orellana J (eds) (1991). Treatment of Retinopathy of Prematurity. Chicago: Year Book-Mosby

McPherson AR, Hittner HM, Kretzer FL (eds) (1986). Retinopathy of Prematurity. Current Concepts and Controversies. Philadelphia: BC Decker

Owens WC, Owens EW (1948). Retrolental fibroplasia in premature infants. Trans Am Acad Ophthalmol Otolaryngol 53:18-41

Patz A, Hoeck LE, De La Cruz E (1952). Studies of the effect of high oxygen administration in retrolental fibroplasia: nursery observations. Am J Ophthalmol 27:1248-1253

Reese AB, Payne J (1946). Persistence and hyperplasia of the primary vitreous: tunica vasculosa lentis or retrolental fibroplasia. Am J Ophthalmol 29:1-24

Terry TL (1942). Extreme prematurity and fibroblastic overgrowth of persistent vascular sheath behind each crystalline lens. I. Preliminary report. Am J Ophthalmol 25:203-204

Figures

FIGURE 18-1.
"Plus disease." Eye of an infant born at 27 weeks after a normal pregnancy, weighing 900 g at birth. Upon examination in the nursery at 10 weeks after birth, we can see dilated arteries and veins as they course to and from the disc. This is an example of "plus disease."

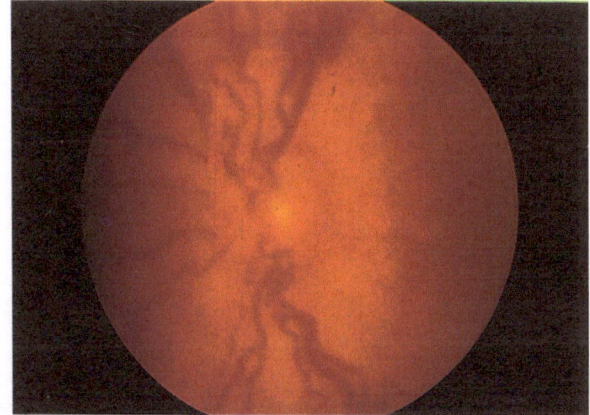

FIGURE 18-2.
Stage 3 disease. Examination of the periphery reveals an arteriovenous shunt with both intraretinal and extraretinal neovascularization. The shunt has height and width.

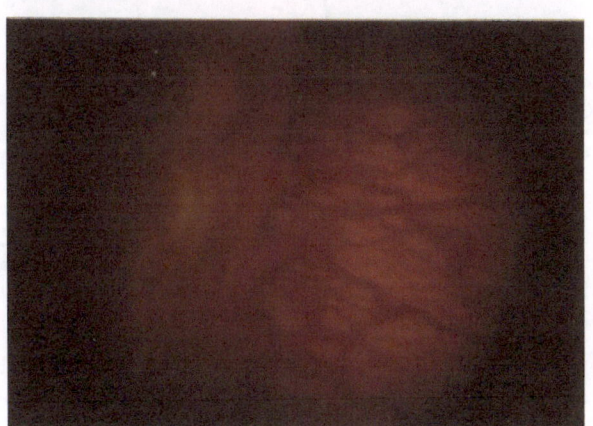

FIGURE 18-3.
Stage 5 disease. The child has total retinal detachment and presented to the office with leukocoria. Open-sky vitrectomy was performed by one of the authors (J.O.). The acuity after 2 years is at the level of count fingers.

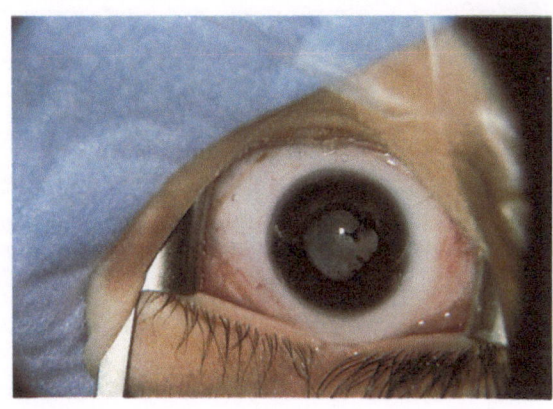

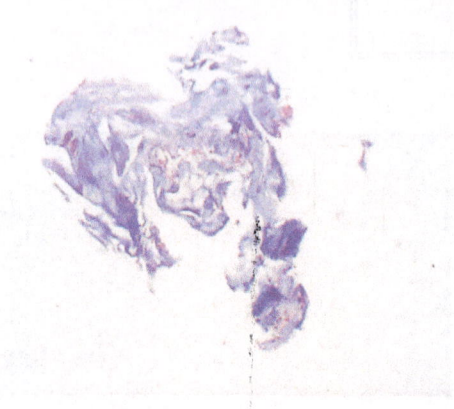

FIGURE 18-4.
Membrane removed at surgery shows extensive collagen with some vascular spaces. The surgery was performed when the child was 1 year old. (Masson-Trichrome) Courtesy of Eichenbaum JW, Mamelok A, Mittl RN, Orellana J (eds) (1991). Treatment of Retinopathy of Prematurity. Chicago: Year Book-Mosby.

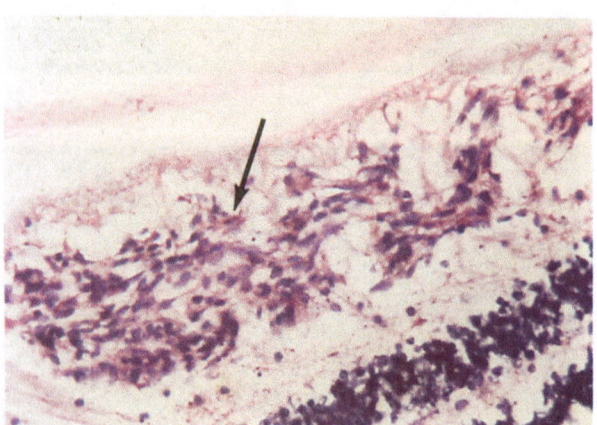

FIGURE 18-5.
Note the endothelial cell proliferation. (H & E) (arrow)

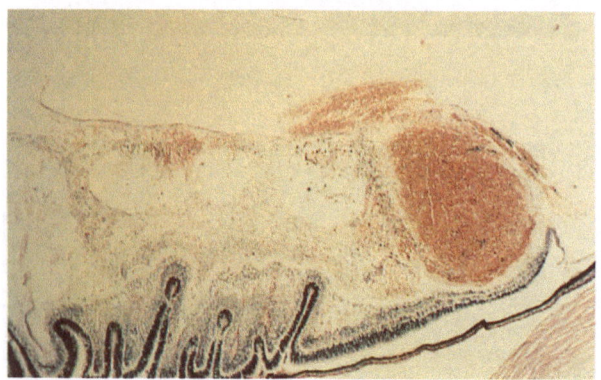

FIGURE 18-6.
Retinal folds and vitreous hemorrhage are evident. (H & E)

FIGURE 18-7.
This patient stated that she had never had vision in her left eye. She remembered being told that she had a total retinal detachment as a child. Acuity in the right eye was 20/70. Although she has a cataract, she exhibits temporal dragging. The macula is displaced inferiotemporally, and there is a macular hole present. She has retrolental fibroplasia, the cicatricial form of retinopathy of prematurity. In the temporal periphery, there were avascular regions with extensive pigmentation.

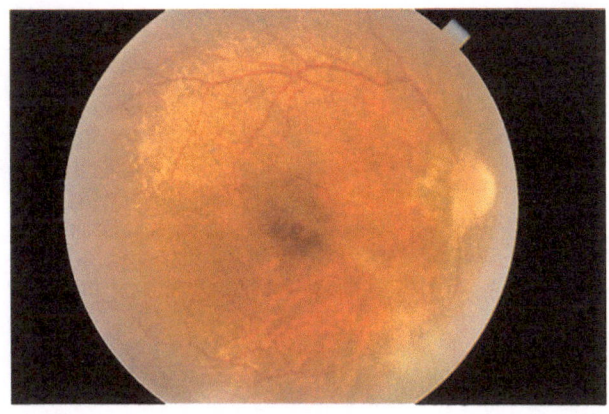

Chapter 19

Sickle Cell Disease

Substitution of the amino acid valine for glutamic acid converts adult hemoglobin (A) to sickle (S) hemoglobin. If lysine is substituted for glutamic acid, hemoglobin C results. Although patients who have a double dose of S hemoglobin develop systemic problems—crisis, anemia, and hemolysis—those with S-C or sickle-thalassemia develop ocular problems. Arterial occlusions and infarction of the optic nerve can be seen. One fourth of patients with S-S disease will have maculopathy.

Proliferative and nonproliferative retinopathy develops in these patients. Black sunbursts (combination of melanin and hemosiderin) and preretinal hemorrhages (salmon patches) appear. The proliferative changes can be staged: The initial stage is peripheral occlusions, the second stage peripheral anastomosis the third stage peripheral neovascularization, and the fourth stage vitreous hemorrhage. The fifth and final stage is retinal detachment.

Therapy is directed at the stage of involvement. Argon laser photocoagulation is indicated for neovascularization (sea fans). Early vitrectomy is advised, as many of these eyes progress easily to traction detachments, which are difficult to repair. Scleral buckling procedures can cause anterior segment ischemia so vitrectomy and segmented buckles are safer in these patients. Histopathologically, vascular occlusions, retinal ischemia, and atrophy are seen. Fibrovascular tissue, as well as chorioretinal atrophy can also be present. Sunbursts characteristically contain hemosiderin-laden macrophages.

Suggested Reading

Clarkson JG (1992). The ocular manifestations of sickle cell disease: A revalence and natural history study. Transactions of the American Ophthalmological Society 90:481-504

Goldberg MF (1971). Classification and pathogenesis of proliferative sickle retinopathy. Am J Ophthalmol 71:649-665

Goldberg MF, Acacio I (1973). Argon laser photocoagulation of proliferative sickle retinopathy. Arch Ophthalmol 90:35-44

Jampol LM, Goldbaum MH (1980). Peripheral proliferative retinopathies. Surv Ophthalmol 25:1-14

Figures

FIGURE 19-1.
Junction between avascular and vascular retina (peripheral occulsions). This picture represents stage 1 disease.

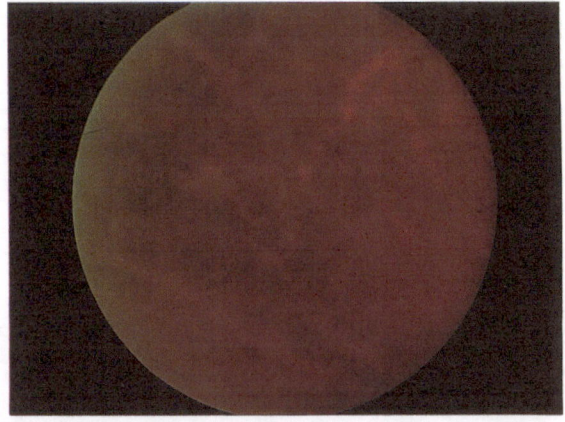

FIGURE 19-2.
Fluorescein angiogram demonstrating the arteriovenous anastomosis developing at this nonperfused area.

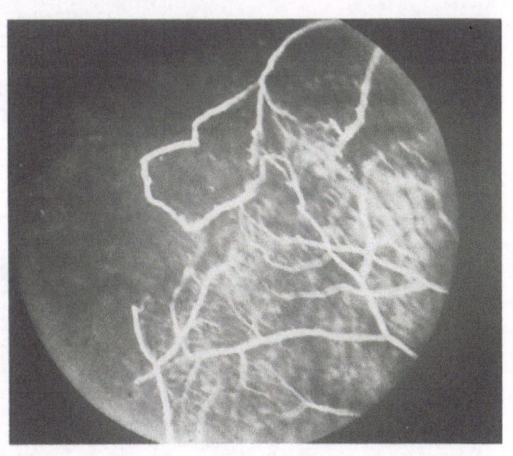

FIGURE 19-3.
Sea-fan formation. It is more commonly seen in SC disease. (Courtesy of Alfred J. Nadel, M.D.)

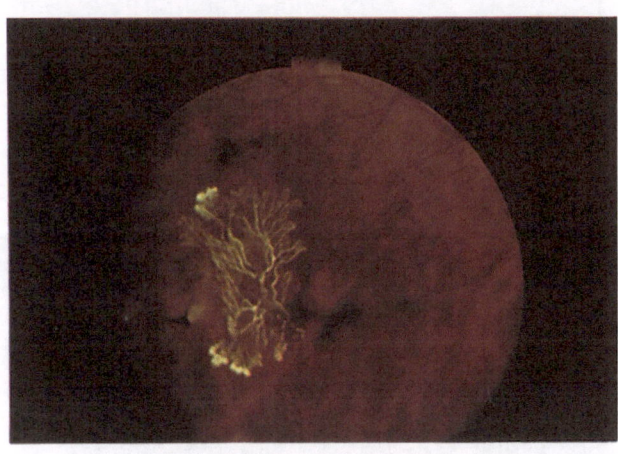

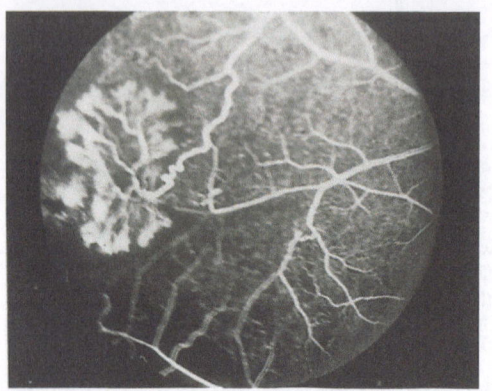

FIGURE 19-4.
Fluorescein angiogram delineating the sea-fan formation. (Courtesy of Alfred J. Nadel, M.D.)

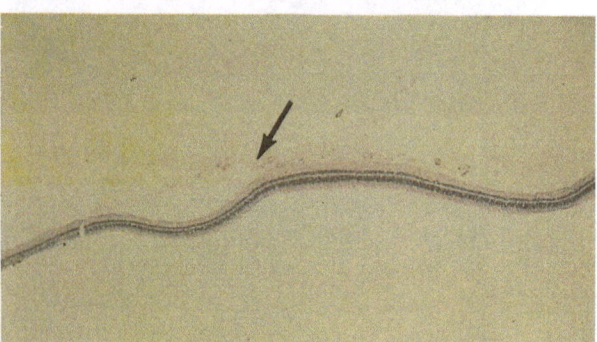

FIGURE 19-5.
Sea-fan. The neovascular tuft leaves the retina and enters the vitreous as a sea-fan. (H & E) (arrow)

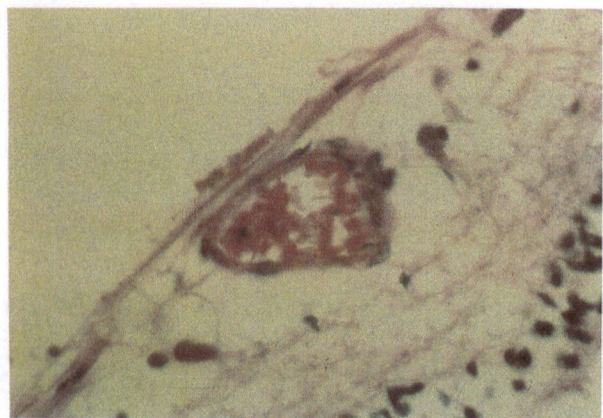

FIGURE 19-6.
Autopsy specimen obtained from a patient who died during a sickle crisis. Sickled cells can be seen in the lumen of the choriocapillaris.

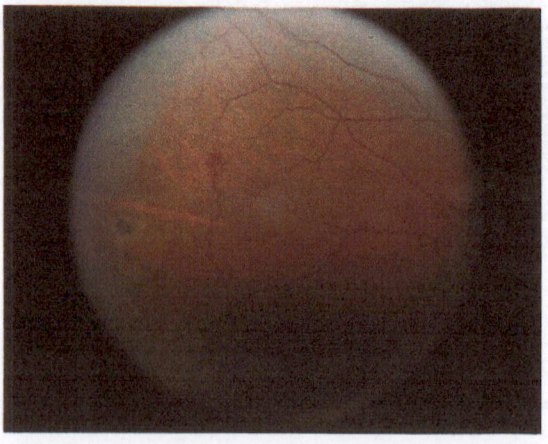

FIGURE 19-7.
Stage III disease. Pigment epithelial hyperplasia can be seen in areas where intraretinal hemorrhages have occurred. A sunburst can be seen at the left. Sunbursts are more commonly seen with SS disease.

Section 5

Vitreous

Chapter 20

Bergmeister's Papilla

The presence of glial tissue on the optic nerve head constitutes the condition commonly known as Bergmeister's papilla, also known as an epipapillary veil. The glial tissue often fills in the optic cup such that the cup is obliterated. The nasal disc appears to be more involved with the glial tissue than is the temporal disc.

Embryologically, the hyaloid vessels are enclosed in a fibrous sheath. Should this sheath not resolve as the hyaloid vessels resolve, the epipapillary veil is left. Hence it is not unusual to see a prepapillary vascular loop in patients with a Bergmeister's papilla.

Visual acuity is not affected. The condition appears to be an incidental finding. Fluorescein angiography is normal. If a prepapillary loop is present, it is evident on the fluorescein angiogram. Electophysiology is normal, as are the visual fields.

Histologically, Bermeister's papilla is glial tissue.

Selected Reading

Bergmeister O (1877). Beiträge zur Entwicklungsgeschichte des Saugethierauges in Shenk SL (ed). Mitteilungen aus dem Embryologischen Institut der Univ Wien: Vol. 1:63-81

Roth AM, Foos RY (1982). Surface structure of the optic nerve head: epipapillary membranes. Am J Ophthalmol 74:977-985

Figures

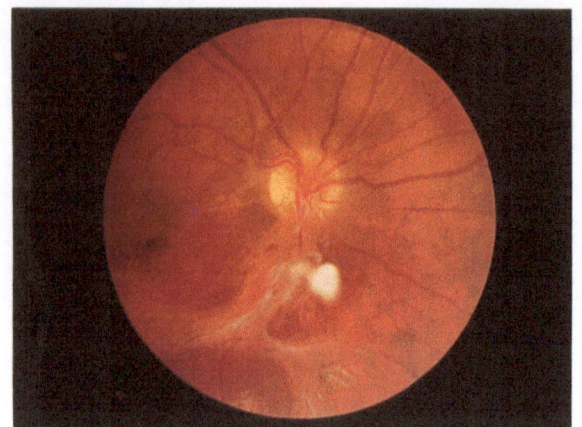

FIGURE 20-1.
There is an exuberant amount of glial tissue on the disc in this patient, with a dense plug of it just inferior to the disc. Acuity remains unaffected. (Courtesy of Marvin Kraushar, M.D.)

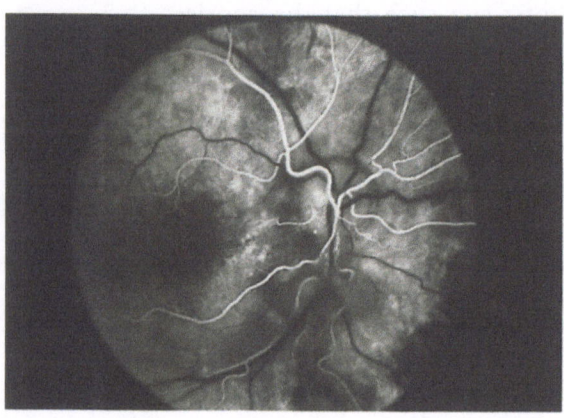

FIGURE 20-2.
Arterial phase fluorescein angiogram demonstrating normal vasculature. The glial tissue can barely be noted, except for the dense gray plug seen inferior to the disc. (Courtesy of Marvin Kraushar, M.D.)

Chapter 21

Persistent Hyaloid Artery

As with Bergmeister's papilla, failure of total reabsorption of the intravitreal portion of the hyaloid system produces a persistent hyaloid artery. In children, as in adults, the vessel does not usually contain blood, and so the risk of hemorrhage is practically nonexistent. Persistence of the hyaloid artery is seen commonly in premature infants and should be kept in mind when performing surgery for stage 5 retinopathy of prematurity. The attachment of the artery to the posterior aspect of the lens is called a Mittendorf dot. Embryologically, the artery enters the posterior lens at this point. Upon atrophy of the artery, the capsule closes, and the arterial system recedes.

No visual abnormalities are seen unless a hyaloid vessel happens to contain blood and ruptures. Severe cases may necessitate vitreous surgery.

Selected Reading

Delaney Jr WV (1980). Prepapillary hemorrhage and persistent hyaloid artery. Am J Ophthalmol 90:419-421

Jack RL (1969). Ultrastructure of the hyaloid vascular system. Arch Ophthalmol 87:555-567

Figures

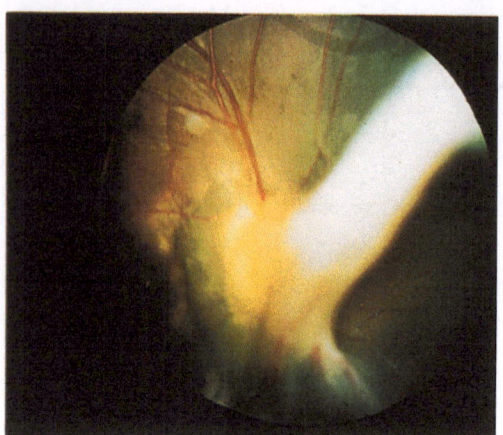

FIGURE 21-1.
Clinical photograph showing a dense hyaloid system emanating from the center of the disc. Hyaloid vessels are present and end as a dot on the posterior aspect of the lens. (Courtesy of Marvin Kraushar, M.D.)

Chapter 22

Persistent Hyperplastic Primary Vitreous

Persistent hyperplastic primary vitreous (PHPV) must be considered in the differential diagnosis of leukocoria. PHPV is unilateral in more than 80% of cases, and bilateral in about 20%. It has a sporadic heredity pattern; that is, no discernible sign of genetic transmission is present, although PHPV has been seen in association with trisomy 13.

Clinically, the condition presents in several ways, depending on the severity and extent of involvement. Embryologically, the primary vitreous recedes as the secondary and ultimately tertiary vitreous become dominant. If the primary vitreous does not recede but remains to a great degree, the condition of PHPV exists. A spectrum of involvement can be seen. Anteriorly, the disease may be limited to invasion of the lens, with subsequent cataract formation. These patients do well with a lensectomy and anterior vitrectomy. In these mild cases there may also be a persistent hyaloid artery, or Bergmeister's papilla. Further involvement of the anterior segment may compromise the uveal structures, producing elongated ciliary processes, peripheral retinal traction, and even microphthalmia. If the tunica vasculosa lentis is still present, it may hinder visual evaluation of the eye.

In more advanced stages, retinal masses may extend from the disc to the retinal periphery. With sufficient anteroposterior traction, extensive retinal detachment can be produced. Other retinal alterations, such as dysplasia and retinal nodules, have been described. Surgery depends on how extensively the eye has been altered by the PHPV. Simple anterior segment involvement may respond to lensectomy, although a peripapillary detachment with multiple folds may not be amenable to vitreoretinal techniques.

Ultrasonography and computed tomography are the best diagnostic methods available. In an older child the evidence of leukocoria and microphthalmia after a normal gestational age birth should bring the diagnosis of PHPV to mind. The absence of intraocular calcification helps rule out retinoblastoma. If the child has glaucoma due to shallowing of the anterior segment, surgery should be performed.

Selected Reading

Blodi FC (1972). Preretinal glial nodules in persistence and hyperplasia of the primary vitreous. Arch Ophthalmol 87:531-534

Federman JL, Shields JA, Altman B, Koller H (1982). The surgical and nonsurgical management of persistent primary vitreous. Ophthalmology 89:20-24

Font RL, Yanoff M, Zimmerman LE (1969). Intraocular adipose tissue and persistent hyperplastic primary vitreous. Arch Ophthalmol 82:43-50

Goldberg MF, Mafee M (1983). Computed tomography for diagnosis of persistent hyperplastic primary vitreous (PHPV). Ophthalmology 90:442-451

Pruett RC (1975). The pleomorphism and complications of posterior hyperplastic primary vitreous. Am J Ophthalmol 80:625-629

Reese AB (1955). Persistent hyperplastic primary vitreous. Am J Ophthalmol 40:317-331

Figures

FIGURE 22-1.
Globe is of normal size in this child with PHPV. The lens is clear, but there is fibrous invasion of the posterior capsule. The tissue located behind the lens is vascularized. Intraocular diathermy must be used to cauterize these vessels before they are severed. Ultrasonography demonstrated that the PHPV was in fact located anteriorly and did not involve the posterior pole.

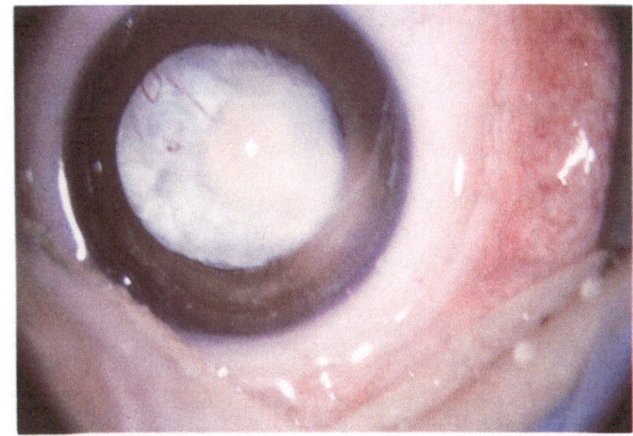

FIGURE 22-2.
Histopathology demonstrates invasion of the posterior aspect of the lens (L) by the fibrous tissue derived from the primary vitreous. (H & E)

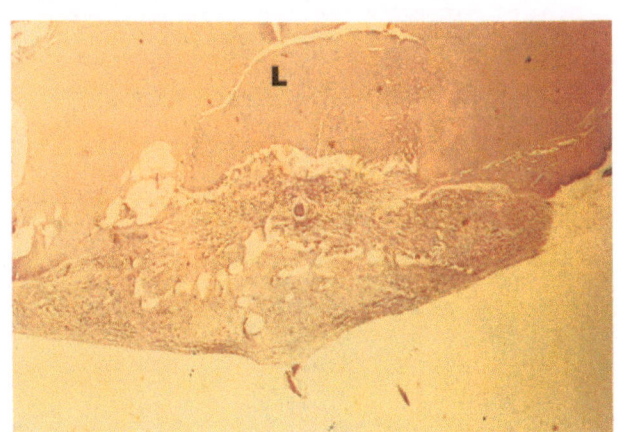

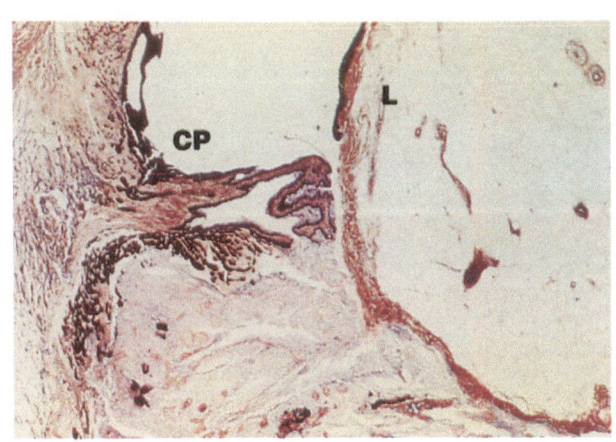

FIGURE 22-3.
Commonly the iris processes are pulled in by the retrolental tissues. In this pathology specimen, the ciliary processes (CP) are compressed and pulled in by the primary vitreous tissue. Note the intralenticular (L) deposit of adipose cells, a characteristic finding in endstage PHPV. (PTAH)

Chapter 23

Pigmented Vitreous Cyst

Intraocular cysts can be seen in both anterior and posterior segments. Originally described in 1899, these cysts are seen with retinitis pigmentosa, uveitis, or chorioretinal atrophy. Many investigators consider the cysts to be congenital in origin, but they may also result from trauma. The pigmented ciliary epithelium may be the source of the cysts.

B-scan ultrasonography will demonstrate the cystic nature of these lesions in the vitreous. All other tests are normal.

Histopathology reveals cuboidal cells with large spheroidal melanin granules. The basement membrane is thin and polarized with numerous microvilli.

Selected Reading

Brewerton EW (1913). Cysts in the vitreous. Trans Ophthalmol Soc UK 33:93-94

Orellana J, O'Malley RE, McPherson AR, Font RL (1985). Pigmented free-floating vitreous cysts in two young adults: electron microscopic observations. Ophthalmology 92:297-302

Sugar HS, Blau RP (1973). Free-floating cysts of the ocular media. Ann Ophthalmol 5:445-453

Tansley JO (1899). Cyst of the vitreous. Trans Am Ophthalmol Soc 5:507-509

Figures

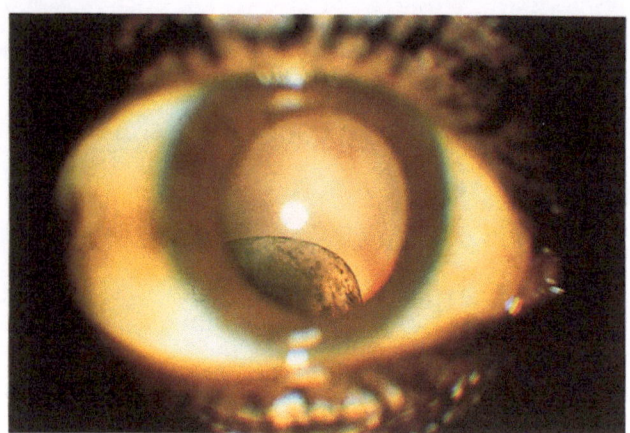

FIGURE 23-1.
The patient noted a gradually enlarging vitreous floater that was mobile. When the pigmented vitreous cyst did not obscure the visual axis, acuity was 20/20.

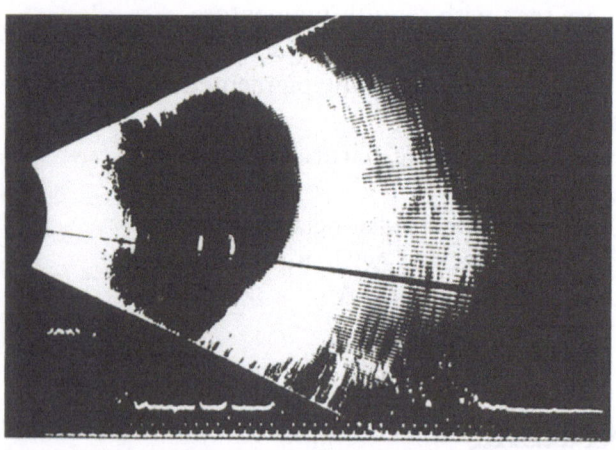

FIGURE 23-2.
Ultrasonography shows the floater to indeed be a cyst.

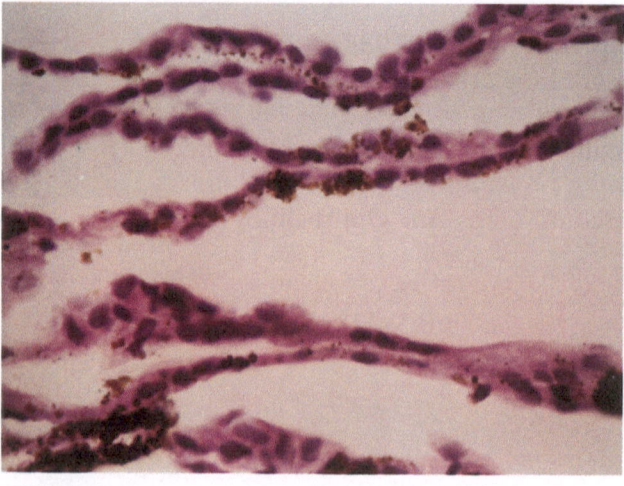

FIGURE 23-3.
Histopathology demonstrates pigment epithelial cells lining the cavity. The pigment granules are large and coarse. (H & E) (From Orellana J, O'Malley RE, McPherson AR, Font RL. Pigmented free-floating vitreous cysts in two young adults: Electron microscopic observations. Ophthalmology 92:297-302, 1985. With permission.)

Section 6

Optic Nerve

Chapter 24

Optic Atrophy

There are several disorders in which optic atrophy plays a prominent role. The genetics vary from one disorder to another. Congenital optic atrophy can be recessive or dominant. Recessive optic atrophy is congenital and rare. It is usually discovered before the child enters school. The electroretinogram (ERG) is normal. Most children are severely visually impaired. Nystagmus is a feature of this disorder.

Dominant optic atrophy is discovered in children usually during the latter part of the first decade. Acuity is reduced but not markedly so. There is nystagmus and a normal visual field to white targets. The patients have an acquired blue-yellow dyschromatopsia, and there is temporal pallor of the disc. The condition progresses.

Another type of optic atrophy (Leber's disease) may stem from the inability to detoxify cyanide. The pattern of heredity is mitochondrial. (Chapter 3) Patients have headaches and vertigo. The patients lose central vision during their twenties. Visual fields depict dense scotomas in the fixational area. The ERG and dark adaptation are normal. The patients go through a neuritis phase before the atrophy develops.

Other optic atrophies are related to heredodegenerative neurological disorders such as Charcot-Marie-Tooth syndrome. Optic atrophy associated with ataxia is called Behr syndrome. These patients have a positive Babinski sign, increased tendon reflexes, ataxia, muscular rigidity, and a positive Romberg sign. Their vision is limited, and they have a central scotoma. The ERG and dark adaptation are normal.

Selected Reading

Kjer P (1959). Infantile optic atrophy with dominant mode of inheritance: a clinical and genetic study of 19 Danish families. Acta Ophthalmol Suppl (Copenh) 54

Sergott RC (1991). Pediatric neuro-ophthalmology. In LB Leonard, JH

Calhoun, RD Harley (eds): Pediatric Ophthalmology. 3rd Ed. Philadelphia: Saunders

Walsh FB, Hoyt WF (1969). Clinical Neuro-ophthalmology. 3rd Ed. Baltimore: Williams & Wilkins

Figures

FIGURE 24-1.
This patient has optic atrophy due to Leber's hereditary optic atrophy. Note how this condition differs from that seen in end-stage glaucoma where the cup is deep and excavated. (Courtesy of Steven Bodine, M.D.)

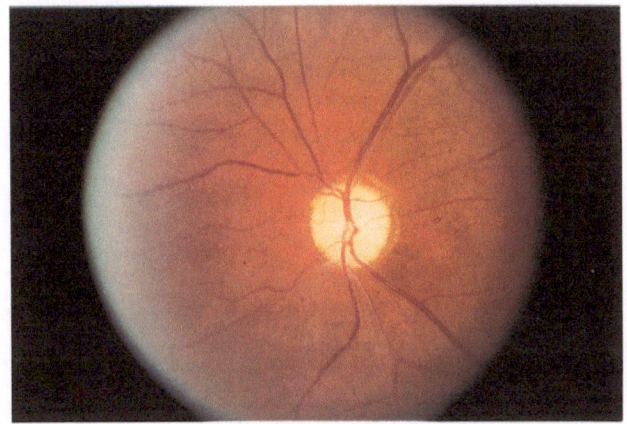

Chapter 25

Ocular Coloboma

The fetal fissure closes in the inferonasal quadrant and may involve the iris, lens, retina, choroid, and optic nerve. Colobomas that involve the anterior segment of the eye may demonstrate a teardrop defect in the inferonasal quadrant of the iris. If the lens is also involved, the zonules in that quadrant may be loose or absent, producing a notch in the lens. Any or all layers of the posterior segment can be affected. Typically, chorioretinal colobomas have a white central defect outlined by pigment epithelium. There may be retina present within the defect, and it is not unusual to see some retinal vessels crossing through the defect. The clinical appearance of a disc coloboma may range from an enlarged and deep cup to a large hole with a retrobulbar cyst. In patients with retinal detachment, it is prudent to investigate for a break along the edge of the coloboma. Ideally, the optimal method for repairing these detachments involves a pars plana vitrectomy with endolaser photocoagulation and internal tamponade with gas or silicone oil.

Colobomas tend to be bilateral. Visual acuity is variable depending on what is affected. Colobomas may be associated with other syndromes, such as trisomy 13 or 18 (cat's eye syndrome). It is autosomal dominant and has variable penetrance. Other genetic syndromes associated with this condition include Lenz's microphthalmos syndrome, Warburg syndrome, and Aicardi syndrome. Deletions and duplications of chromosomal arms may also be associated with colobomas.

Fluorescein angiography demonstrates a defect corresponding to the coloboma. Visual field evaluation reveals a defect that also corrresponds to the coloboma's extent and location. Color vision may be abnormal; and depending on the size of the coloboma, the electroretinogram and electroculogram may also be abnormal.

Histologically, the choroid is atrophied or simply absent; there is no retinal pigment epithelium, and the retina is gliotic. Examination of the section may reveal the presence of rosettes. The edges of the coloboma are lined with hyperplastic pigment epithelium, and the sclera is generally thin. In patients with a disc coloboma and choristoma, the eyes are microophthalmic with fat tissue and smooth muscle next to, or part of, the disc.

Selected Reading

Font RL, Zimmerman LE (1971). Intrascleral smooth muscle in coloboma of the optic disk: electron microscopic verification. Am J Ophthalmol 72:452-457

Gopal L, Kini MM, Sengamedu SS, Sharma T (1991). Management of retinal detachment with choroidal coloboma. Ophthalmology 98:1622-1627

Jesberg DO, Schepens CL (1961). Retinal detachment associated with coloboma of the choroid. Arch Ophthalmol 65:163-173

Pagon RA (1981). Ocular coloboma. Surv Ophthalmol 25:223-236

Figures

FIGURE 25-1.
Colobomas may exist anywhere in the inferonasal quadrant along the fetal fissure. This youth has an iris coloboma. The lens is suspended from the lens fibers. Colobomas may involve the lids, iris, lens, choroid, retina, or optic nerve singly or in combination.

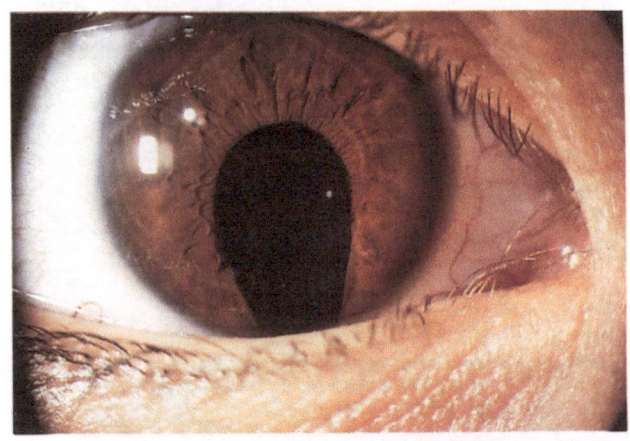

FIGURE 25-2.
Retinochoroidal coloboma. The defect is white, most likely due to glial tissue. The vessels exit the disc, and the margins of the coloboma are hyperpigmented. In children with such a coloboma and a retinal detachment, the break should be sought at the margins of the coloboma.

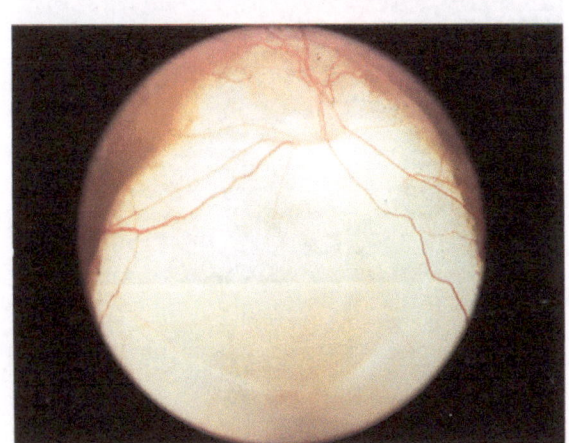

FIGURE 25-3.
Colobomatous disc with a proliferation of the intercalary membrane, that is, glial tissue. This child also had extra rows of eyelashes.

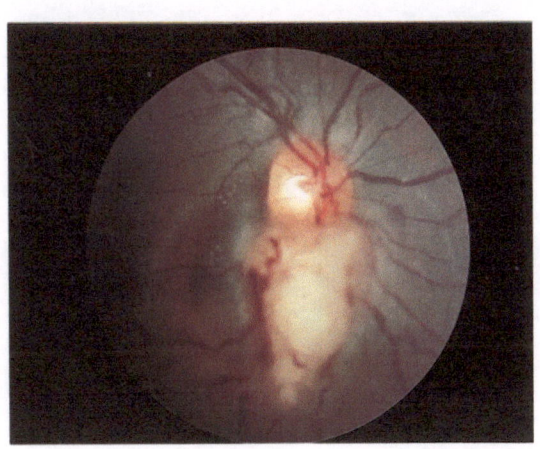

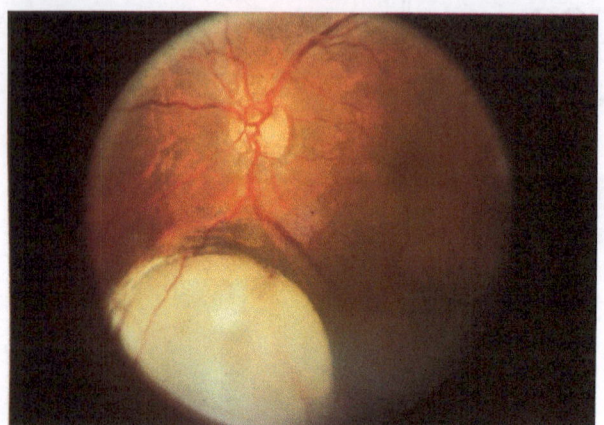

FIGURE 25-4.
Optic disc that appears normal. The coloboma is situated away from the disc and involves the inferonasal quadrant only. The fluorescein angiogram for this eye can be seen in Fig. 4-14.

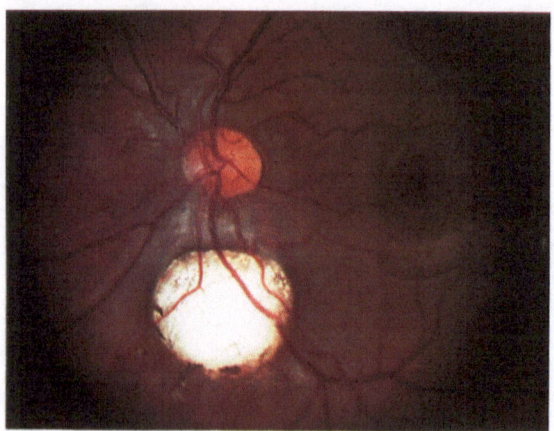

FIGURE 25-5.
Disc appears normal. Inferiorly, a retinal coloboma can be seen, with some pigment cells within it. The fellow eye has an identical coloboma.

Chapter 26

Drusen of the Optic Nerve

It is not unusual to see patients evaluated for papilledema when in fact they have optic nerve drusen. Three patients in 1000 demonstrate drusen of the optic nerve. In familial cases, the inheritance is autosomal dominant. These patients may be asymptomatic or may note a decrease in visual acuity (25%). Visual field defects are seen in 25% of the patients. Drusen are rare in oriental or black persons. Clinical evaluation may demonstrate an irregular nerve head with multiple excrescences on the surface. Because many cases have the drusen deep within the nerve, blurring of the margins of the disc may be all that is present. At times, the drusen grow; and if they are located adjacent to a vessel, optic atrophy, optic nerve hemorrhage, juxtapapillary subretinal hemorrhages, or an infarct may ensue. In cases where one suspects buried drusen, computed tomography and B-scan ultrasonography may be helpful.

Histopathological evaluation reveals ocular, frequently calcified, concentric laminations.

Selected Reading

Acers TE (1983). Congenital Abnormalities of the Optic Nerve and Related Forebrain. Philadelphia: Lea & Febiger

Friedman AH, Beckerman B, Gold DH, Walsh JB (1977). Drusen of the optic disc. Surv Ophthalmol 21:375-390

Lorentzen SE (1966). Drusen of the optic disc: a clinical and genetic study. Acta Ophthalmol Suppl (Copenh) 90

Figures

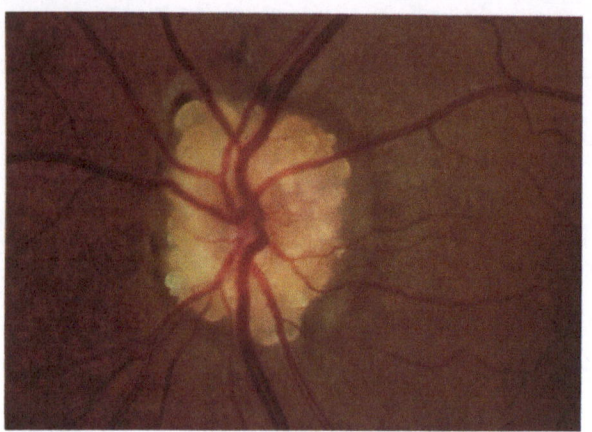

FIGURE 26-1.
Multiple crystalline deposits in the prelaminar level of the nerve head. The patient had originally been referred to rule-out papilledema.

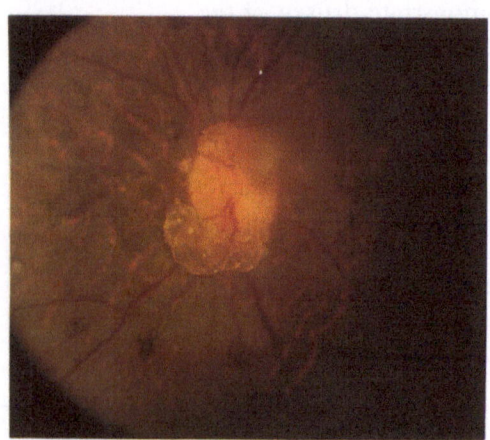

FIGURE 26-2.
Drusen of the optic nerve head and retinitis pigmentosa. Curiously, the patient noted the inferonasal loss of field (typically seen) before any other symptom of the retinitis pigmentosa was evident.

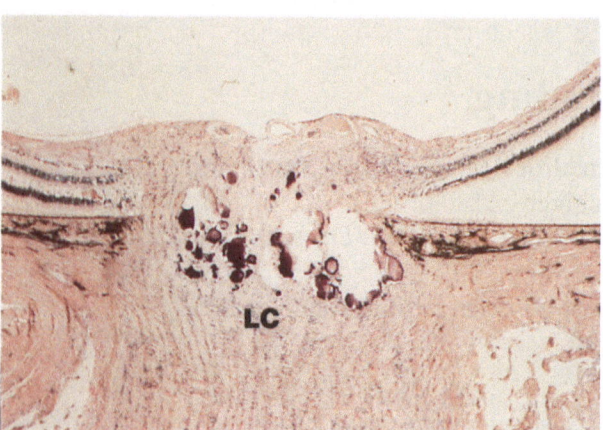

FIGURE 26-3.
Histopathological examination of this optic nerve reveals multiple drusen anterior to the lamina cribrosa. (LC) (H & E)

Chapter 27

Optic Nerve Hypoplasia and Megalopapilla

Optic Nerve Hypoplasia

Children with optic nerve hypoplasia may have multiple endocrine and central nervous system problems. The discs in these patients have fewer nerve fibers than normal, and there is a deficiency of the retinal ganglion cells. There have been reports of anencephaly and hydranencephaly. De Morsier syndrome has also been described in patients with optic nerve hypoplasia. De Morsier syndrome patients have an absence of the septum pellucidum, partial or complete agenesis of the corpus callosum, pituitary dysfunction, and dysplasia of the third ventricle. Apert syndrome and Meckel syndrome are two other conditions in which optic nerve hypoplasia may coexist. There may be an association with maternal ingestion of quinine, phenytoin, lysergic acid diethylamide (LSD), meperidine, and diuretics as well. It can also be seen in children of diabetic mothers.

Optic nerve hypoplasia can occur unilaterally or bilaterally. Typically, the disc is pale with a surrounding yellow to white ring—the "double ring" sign. Foveal reflexes are poor, and acuity may range from 20/20 to no light perception.

Only ultrasonography is helpful in the office. The B-scan demonstrates small optic nerves. Tomography demonstrates small optic canals. It is interesting to note that, although there are reports of optic nerve aplasia in the literature, many of these cases actually represent instances of optic nerve hypoplasia. Genetic inheritance is sporadic, and the electrophysiological tests depend on the extent of ocular involvement.

Megalopapilla

Megalopapilla is the term assigned to the entity wherein the optic disc is enlarged. It usually appears unilaterally, and the globe is of normal size. Acuity is generally normal, although a slight decrease has been reported.

Systemic associations are cleft palate and encephalocoele. If an encephalocoele is suspected, the best diagnostic tool is computed tomography. The visual field may demonstrate an enlarged blind spot due to the increase in size of the optic disc. No hereditary pattern has been established.

Selected Reading

Acers TE (1981). Optic nerve hypoplasia: septo-optic-pituitary dysplasia syndrome. Trans Am Ophthalmol Soc 79:425-457

Franeschetti A, Bock RH (1950). Megalopapilla: a new congenital anomaly. Am J Ophthalmol 33:227-235

Petersen RA, Walton DS (1977). Optic nerve hypoplasia with good visual acuity and visual field defects: a study of children of diabetic mothers. Arch Ophthalmol 95:254-258

Skarf B, Hoyt CS (1984). Optic nerve hypoplasia in children: association with anomalies of the endocrine and CNS. Arch Ophthalmol 102:62-67

Figures

FIGURE 27-1.
This child presented with de Morsier syndrome, or septo-optic dysplasia. These children have an absence of the septum pellucidum, pituitary insufficiency, and optic nerve hypoplasia. There is failure of the retinal ganglion cells to develop normally. Note the double ring sign present at the optic nerve.

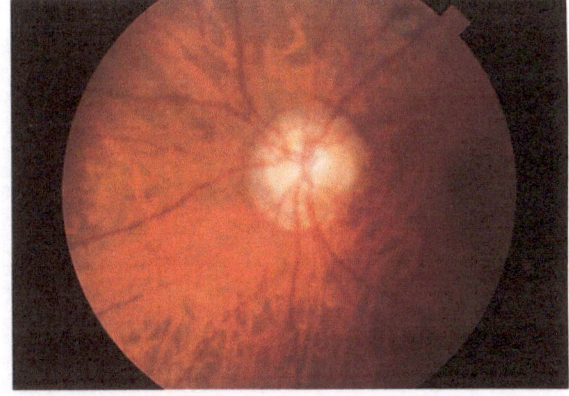

FIGURE 27-2.
Coronal calotte showing the relatively small size of the disc compared to the rest of the retina.

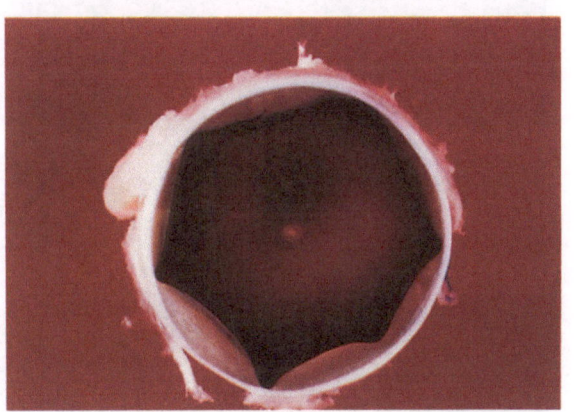

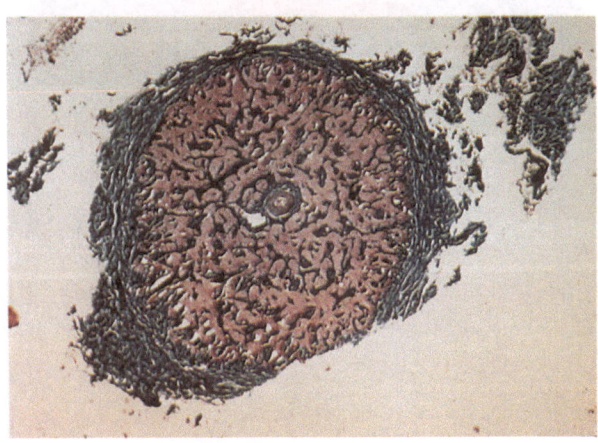

FIGURE 27-3.
Histopathologically, this nerve shows a paucity of neuronal elements with thickened pial septae. (Masson-trichrome)

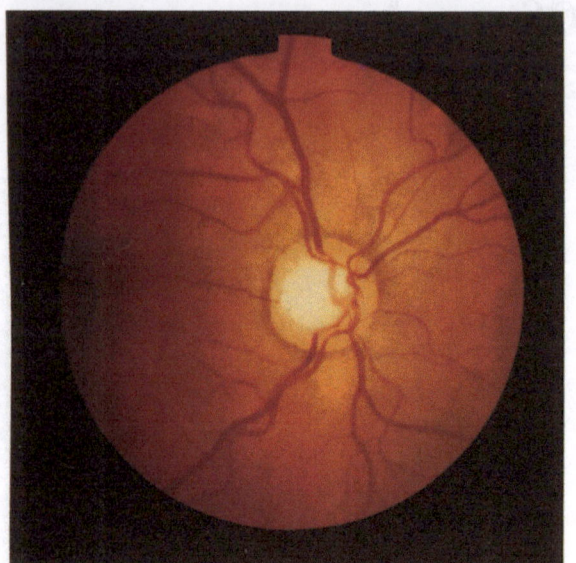

A

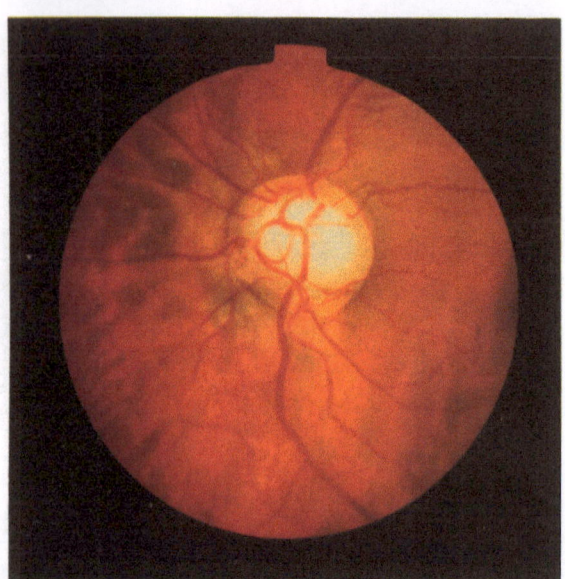

B

FIGURE 27-4.
(A) Normal right eye. (B) Megalopapilla. Note that the optic disc is enlarged.

Chapter 28

Morning Glory Disc Anomaly

It is believed that morning glory discs arise from abnormal development of the posterior sclera during gestation. One hypothesis suggests that the disc and surrounding tissue prolapse posteriorly as a result of failure of the embryological fissure to close. The anomaly resembles a morning glory flower, from which the name was derived. The disc is enlarged, with a core of glial tissue in its center. Around the disc is found altered pigment epithelium. The arteries may be sheathed, and the vasculature appears to emanate radially from the disc. Visual acuity in these eyes is limited to no better than 20/200 in most cases. Many of the patients present with strabismus. Because the disease is unilateral, patching therapy may be helpful to fulfill the visual potential of the affected eye. The condition is found more commonly in females.

Associated ocular findings include microphthalmos, anterior chamber anomalies, and cataracts. There is an associated retinal detachment rate of 30% in these patients. Usually, as with detachments in colobomas, the break is small and located posteriorly around the disc. It is interesting to note that studies have suggested that the subretinal fluid in these patients is actually subarachnoid cerebrospinal fluid. There is no evidence for a characteristic hereditary pattern.

Selected Reading

Apple DJ, Rabb MF, Walsh PM (1982). Congenital anomalies of the optic disc. Surv Ophthalmol 27:3-41

Beyer WB, Quencer RM, Osher RH (1982). Morning glory syndrome: a functional analysis including fluorescein angiography, ultrasonography, and computerized tomography. Ophthalmology 89:1362-1367

Kindler P (1970). Morning glory syndrome: unusual congenital optic disk anomaly. Am J Ophthalmol 69:376-384

Steinkuller PG (1980). The morning glory disc anomaly: case report and literature review. J Pediatr Ophthalmol Strabismus 17:81-95

Von Fricken MA, Dhungel R (1984). Retinal detachments in the morning glory syndrome. Retina 4:97-99

Figures

FIGURE 28-1.
Typical morning glory disc. The center of the disc has a fibroglial core of tissue with the vasculature emanating from the disc. A peripapillary chorioretinal atrophic ring is evident.

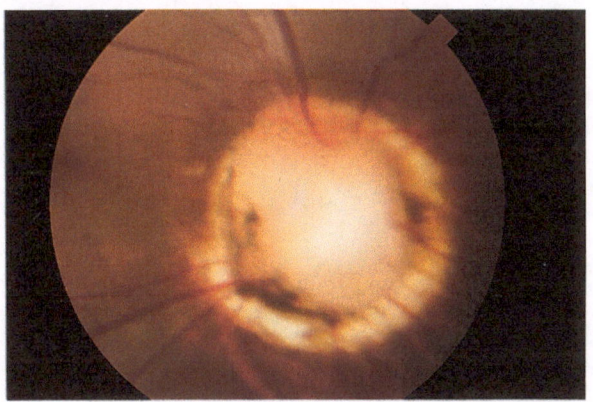

Chapter 29

Congenital Optic Pit

Optic pits occur unilaterally more than 80% of the time. The incidence of optic nerve pits is 1:11,000. The optic pit probably has a sporadic hereditary pattern, although some investigators have suggested that it may be autosomal dominant. Characteristically, the pit is located on the inferotemporal aspect of the disc and may be associated with development of serous detachment of the macula. Optic pits can be slitlike, polygonal or oblong. They can be up to one diopter in depth and .3 disc diameter in width. The latter is usually seen in patients between the ages of 20 and 40. It has been postulated that the fluid is cerebrospinal fluid that has leaked around the nerve sheaths and settled under the macula. The disc abutting the pit has peripapillary atrophy. It is through this area that some investigators believe liquefied vitreous seeps under the macula to create the nonrhegmatogenous detachments. These detachments occur up to 40% of the time. Various visual field defects can be seen, such as an enlarged blind spot, nasal steps, arcuate scotomas, paracentral scotomas, centrocecal scotomas or generalized constriction. The fluorescein angiogram will demonstrate the serous maculopathy, if present. The optic pit exhibits a hyperfluoresence that fades in the late phases.

Accompanying neurological diseases include agenesis of the corpus callosum and encephalocoele. Therapy may be directed at the serous detachment using laser photocoagulation. In long-standing cases, vitrectomy with fluid-air exchange is occasionally beneficial. Histologically, the pit contains neuroectodermal tissue. Other tissues can be found herniated into the optic nerve substance through the pit.

Selected Reading

Brown GC, Shields JA, Goldberg RE (1980). Congenital pits of the optic nervehead. II. Clinical studies in humans. Ophthalmology 87:51-65

Kranenburg EW (1860). Crater-like holes in the optic disc and central serous retinopathy. Arch Ophthalmol 64:912-924

Figures

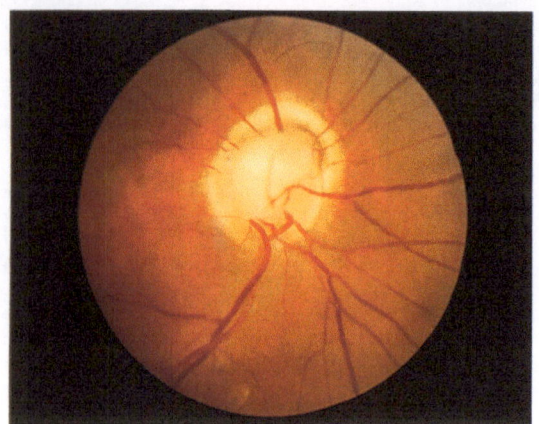

FIGURE 29-1.
Large centrotemporal optic pit. Pits are usually unilateral.

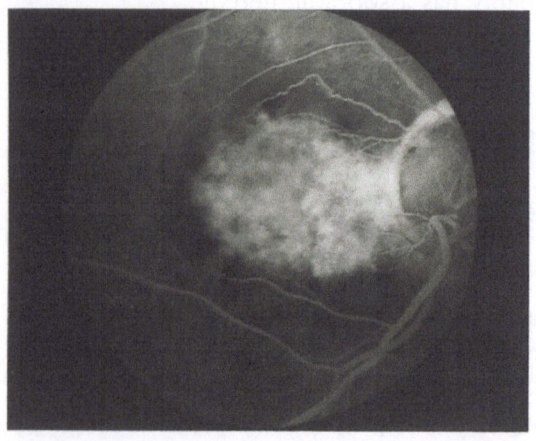

FIGURE 29-2.
Fluorescein angiogram demonstrating that the patient in Fig. 29-1 has an associated serous detachment of the macula.

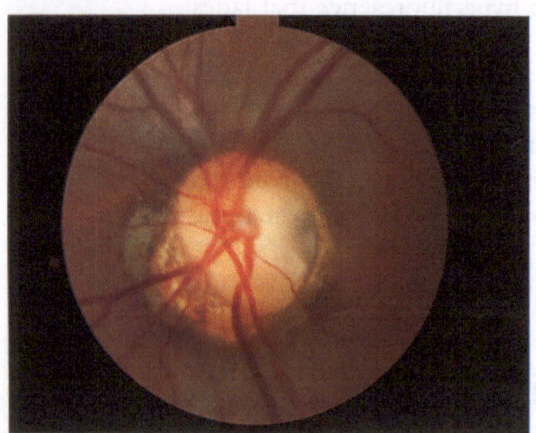

FIGURE 29-3.
Characteristic pit located at the 3 o'clock position. The patient is a 45-year-old woman whose visual acuity is 20/20.

FIGURE 29-4.
Histopathology of an eye with an optic pit shows the depth of this pit in relation to the rest of the optic nerve. The pit is filled with neuroectodermal tissue. (H & E)

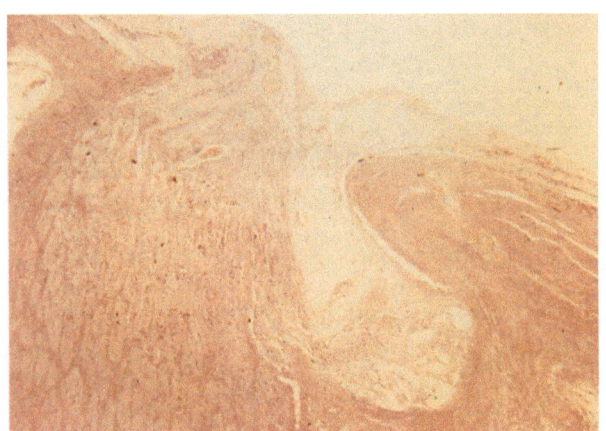

Chapter 30

Tilted Disc

The optic nerve can enter the globe at any angle, and the angulation of the scleral canal can produce a horizontal or vertical malformation. Typically, the horizontal malformation produces the disc configuration seen with myopia, whereas vertical malformation produces the inferior conus or tilted disc configuration. Typically, the retina lies directly touching the sclera in a crescentic area below the disc. Because the disc is at an angle in the scleral canal, the vessels angle upward as they exit the disc in the eye. The disc is tilted inferiorly in two-thirds of cases. Situs inversus of the vascular system is seen in more than three-fourths of the cases. Myopic refraction and often excessive astigmatism is present and most cases are bilateral.

The visual fields show a defect in the superotemporal quadrant, with the defect crossing the midline. Fluorescein angiography can document the absence of papilledema. The presence or absence of papilledema could cause confusion when the examining physician sees no clear disc margins. There can be a diminished electroretinogram. A hereditary pattern has not been demonstrated. Histopathology resembles a typical coloboma, with which it is occassionly associated.

Selected Reading

Dorrell D (1978). The tilted disc. Br J Ophthalmol 62:16-20

Riise D (1966). Visual field defects in optic disc malformation with ectasia of the fundus. Acta Ophthalmologica (Copenh) 44:906-918

Figures

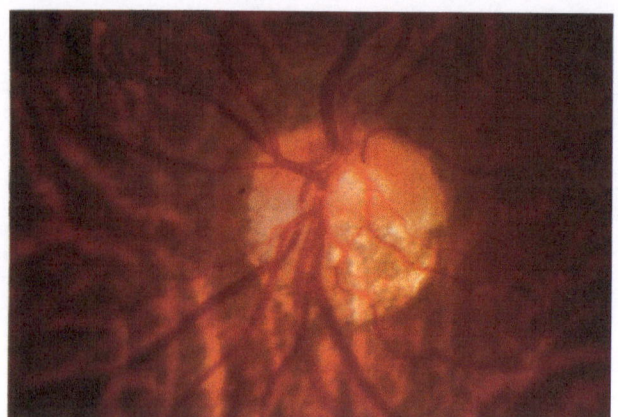

FIGURE 30-1.
Oval discs are not unusual. There is a defect seen inferiorly—a conus or crescent. The vessels are all present, but there may be a primary defect in the retinal pigment epithelium. This patient had a field defect and reduced visual acuity.

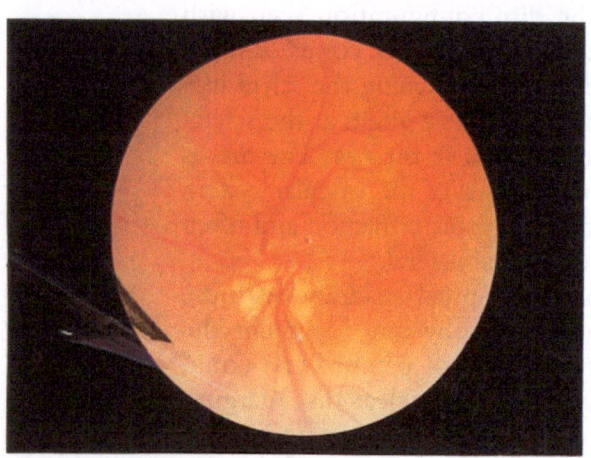

FIGURE 30-2.
This patient also has an inferior nasal-tilted disc. There is a blond fundus present and situs inversus of the exiting vasculature.

Chapter 31

Prepapillary Vascular Loop

A sporadic frequently autosomal dominant anomaly, prepapillary vascular loop appears to be unrelated to the hyaloid artery system, yet it is located on the surface of the disc. It is believed that the loops begin to form during the middle trimester, at which time they are supported by the disc glial tissue. The configuration of these vessels can be a loop, a corkscrew, or a figure eight. The loops arise above the level of the disc for only a short distance and then return to the disc. Most are arterial, and many supply a branch retinal artery. On ocassion, thrombosis of the loop produces amaurosis, vitreous hemorrhage or even hyphema.

Fluorescein angiography demonstrates whether the loops are arterial or venous and if there is any relation to a cilioretinal artery. All other tests are negative. Histopathology demonstrates vessels without an internal elastic lamina.

Selected Reading

Bisland T (1953). Vascular loops in the vitreous. Arch Ophthalmol 49:514-529

Brucker AJ, Michels RG, Fine SL (1977). Congenital retinal arterial loops and vitreous hemorrhage. Am J Ophthalmol 84:220-223

Degenhart W, Brown GC, Augsburger JJ, Magargal LE (1981). Prepapillary vascular loops. Ophthalmology 88:1126-1131

Figures

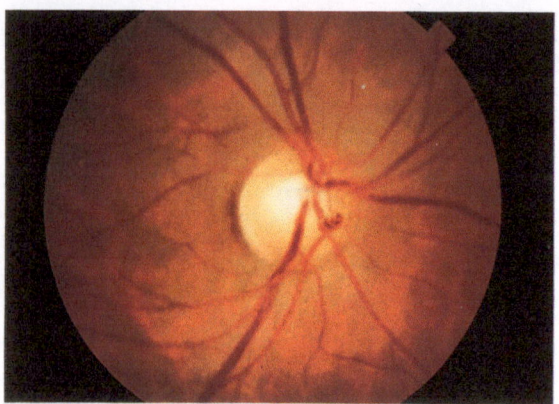

FIGURE 31-1.
A coiled vascular loop can be seen at the optic nerve head.

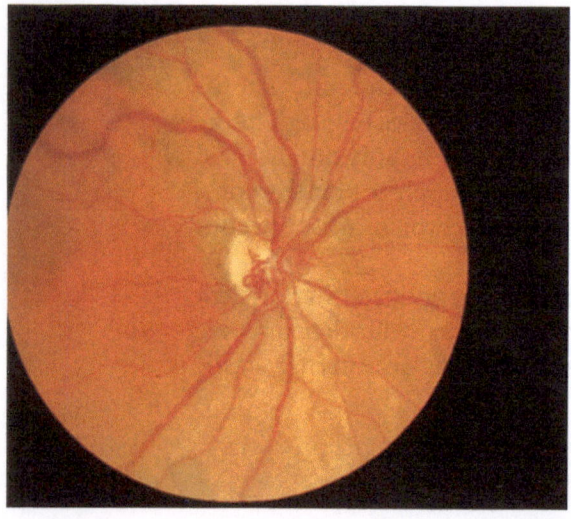

FIGURE 31-2.
Vascular loops in this patient resemble a figure eight. The child was referred because the general ophthalmologist thought the vascular loop was a collection of shunt vessels on the disc.

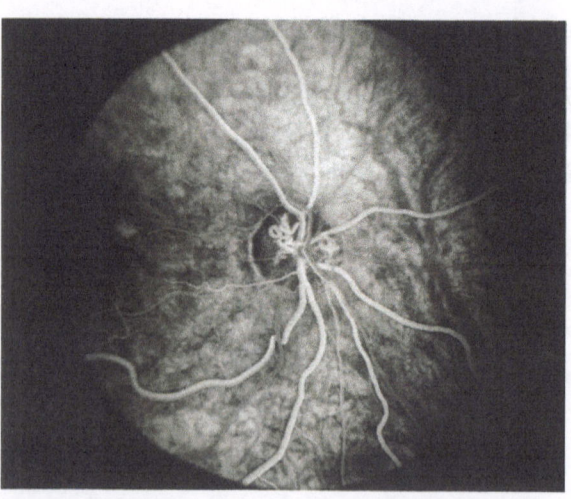

FIGURE 31-3.
Fluorescein angiography demonstrates the vessels on the nerve head.

Section 7

Pigment Epithelium

Chapter 32

Best's Disease

Generalized disease of the retinal pigment epithelium (RPE) seems to be the central problem in patients with Best's disease. This entity is also known as congenital macular dystrophy, vitelliform macular dystrophy, Best's familial macular degeneration, hereditary macular pseudocysts, and hereditary vitelliruptive macular degeneration. It is an autosomal dominant, bilateral condition.

It appears to evolve through stages. Initially, the RPE becomes somewhat bronze in color and evolves into a subretinal "egg yolk" lesion in the fovea. The patient may or may not be asymptomatic at this time. Typically, there is mild visual loss. The lesion may remain stable for many years, with stabilization of acuity. The cystic lesion then undergoes a change, a granular transformation. The vitelliform cyst breaks up into the "scrambled egg" stage. Acuity decreases when the lesion ruptures or resorbs, leaving an oval area of RPE atrophy.

Many of these patients are hyperopic and have a normal visual field. Some patients have a central scotoma. Dark adaptation is normal, and the fluorescein angiogram depends on the stage. When the yellow "yolk" substance is present, the material blocks the fluorescein. During the late stages a central window defect is seen that corresponds to the RPE atrophy at the macula. The electroretinogram is characteristically normal, but the electrooculogram (EOG) is abnormal, which supports the theory that the disease affects the RPE in a broad manner. The EOG is abnormal even in the carriers, who have no evidence of the disease. Thus if a patient with a vitelliform lesion has a normal EOG, a fluorescein angiogram should be performed. If the latter demonstrates increased capillary permeability around the macula, a pseudovitelliform lesion and Best's disease may be ruled out. Genetically, the patients should be counseled that a mild disease in them does not necessarily forecast a mild disease in their offspring. Transmission is autosomal dominant.

Histologically, the RPE cells seem to be primarily involved. The cells demonstrate engorgement and enlargement by lipofuscin granules. The macula demonstrates photoreceptor atrophy.

147

Selected Reading

Best F (1905). Über eine hereditare maculaaffektion: Beiträge zur vererbungslehre. Z Augenheilkd 13:199-212

Fishman GA, Trimble S, Rabb MF, et al (1977). Pseudovitelliform macular dystrophy. Arch Ophthalmol 95:73-76

Kraushar MF, Margolis S, Morse PH, et al (1982). Pseudohypopyon in Best's vitelliform macular dystrophy. Am J Ophthalmol 94:30-37

Schwartz LJ, Metz HS, Woodward F (1972). Electrophysiologic and fluorescein studies in vitelliform macular degeneration. Arch Ophthalmol 87:636-641

Weingeist TA, Kobrin JL, Watzke RC (1982). Histopathology of Best's macular dystrophy. Arch Ophthalmol 100:1108-1114

Figures

FIGURE 32-1.
This patient presented to his ophthalmologist for a routine examination. On funduscopic evaluation, the "egg yolk" appearance was noted in the macula.

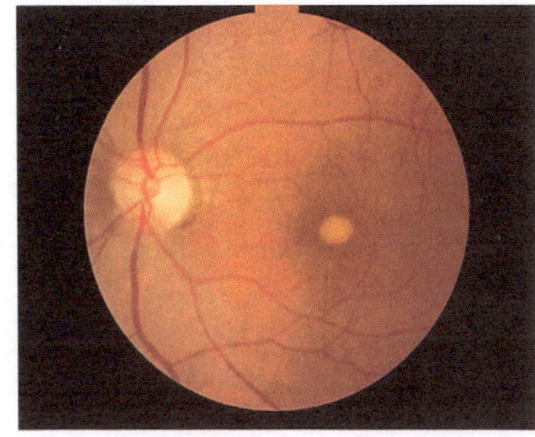

FIGURE 32-2.
"Scrambled egg" appearance of the macula has become prominent in this patient. The cavity has the yellow material layering on the bottom. Acuity in this eye is 20/20.

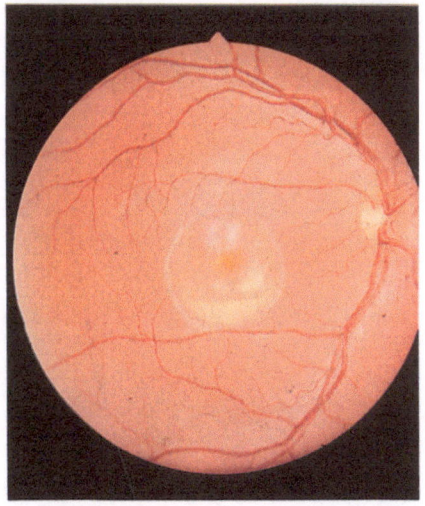

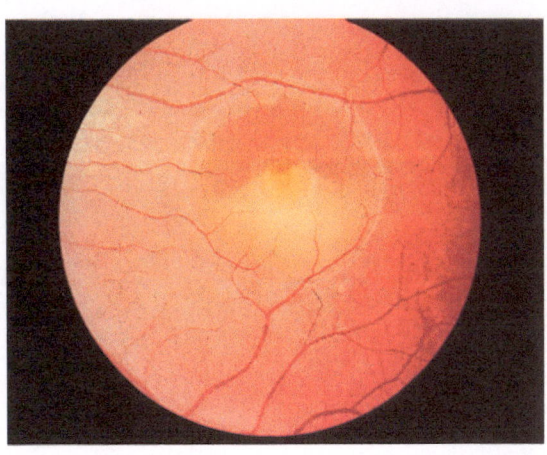

FIGURE 32-3.
Vitelliform lesion occupies most of the cavity in this patient, although the acuity remains 20/30.

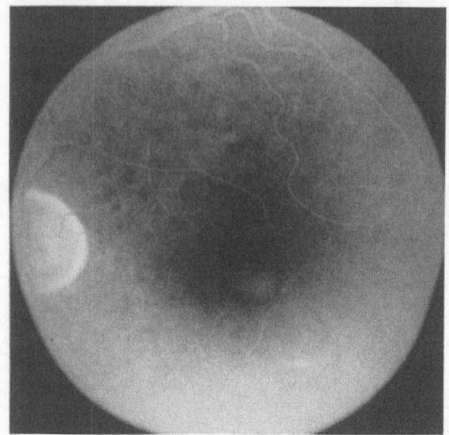

FIGURE 32-4.
Angiogram shows minimal fluorescence and typically the pseudofluorescence of a vitelliform lesion.

Chapter 33

Combined Hamartoma of the Retina and Retinal Pigment Epithelium

Hamartomas of the pigment epithelium are not unusual, especially when the patient has other evidence of congenital malformations. There is usually visual loss. Strabismus or leukocoria may also be a presenting sign. Most diagnoses are made during routine examination of the patient. If the disc-macula is involved directly or by traction, acuity is diminished. Peripheral lesions may not affect the acuity.

Most hamartomas contain tissue elements of pigment epithelium, glial cells, and vascular tissue. Usually one of these tissue types predominates in the lesion. Fluorescein angiography shows hypofluorescence if there is a predominance of pigment epithelial tissue. Vessel distortion and anomalies are clearly delineated as the angiogram progresses. If glial tissue predominates, the lesion may resemble an epiretinal membrane. It must be remembered that a hamartoma does not peel like an epiretinal membrane if vitrectomy and membranectomy (which is definitely not recommended) is performed.

Histopathologically, this entity consists mostly of intraretinal retinal pigment epithelium hyperplasia and abnormal retinal blood vessels.

Selected Reading

Font RL, Moura RA, Shetlar DJ, et al (1989). Combined hamartoma of sensory retina and retinal pigment epithelium. Retina 9:302-311

Gass JDM (1973). An unusual hamartoma of the pigment epithelium and retina simulating choroidal melanoma and retinoblastoma. Trans Am Ophthalmol Soc 71:171-185

Palmer ML, Carney MD, Combs JL (1990). Combined hamartomas of the retinal pigment epithelium and retina. Retina 10:33-36

Figures

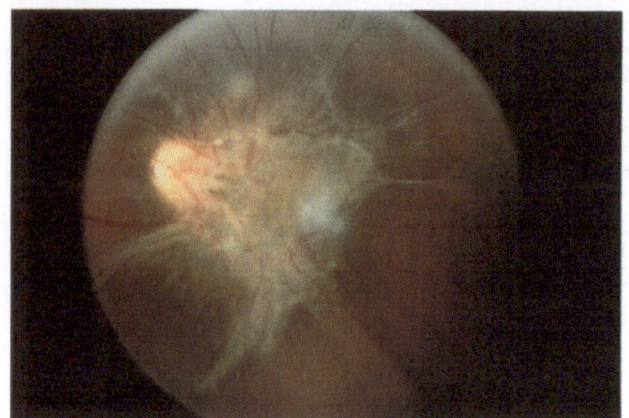

FIGURE 33-1.
This lesion is located mostly juxtapapillary. Characteristically, these lesions are seen in men between the ages of 25 and 40. The lesion is a grayish mass with irregular pigmentation. The macula is involved, and the acuity in this patient is at the hand motions level.

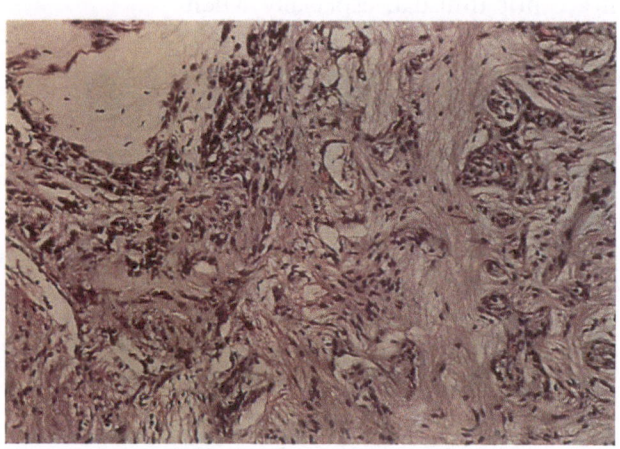

FIGURE 33-2.
Histopathology demonstrates disorganized glial tissue intermingled with vascular tissue and retinal pigment epithelial tubules. (H & E) (Courtesy of Ramon L. Font, M.D.)

Chapter 34

Congenital Hypertrophy of the Retinal Pigment Epithelium

Congenital hypertrophy of the retinal pigment epithelium usually occurs as a solitary lesion, although the lesions can occur in groups. They are black or gray-brown and in young patients are easily identified because of a depigmented "halo" that surrounds the lesion. The lesion is usually round, although it can be oval, and for the most part is flat. As the individual ages, the pigmentation atrophies; usually the black pigment loses its color, leaving a lesion that ultimately becomes round and centrally depigmented. There is often a "halo" of depigmentation around the lesion.

These lesions often occur in groups and have been described as appearing similar to "bear tracks." There appears to be an association with Gardner syndrome (polyposis of the intestines and skeletal hamartomas), angioid streaks and Favre's syndrome.

Fluorescein angiography demonstrates hypofluorescence due to the hyperpigmentation. In regions where there is a depigmented lacuna within the lesion, a normal choriocapillary flush is observed. All electrophysiological testing is normal. A scotoma may be present on visual field examination. The lesion must be distinguished from a hemorrhage under the pigment epithelium, a choroidal nevus, or a choroidal melanoma.

Histologically, there is hypertrophy of the pigment cells with an increase in their melanin content. There may also be a thickening of Bruch's membrane.

Selected Reading

Buettner H (1975). Congenital hypertrophy of the retinal pigment epithelium. Am J Ophthalmol 79:177-189

Cleary PE, Gregor Z, Bird AC (1976). Retinal vascular changes in congenital hypertrophy of the retinal pigment epithelium. Br J Ophthalmol 60:499-507

Lewis RA, Crowder WE, Eierman LA, et al (1984). The Gardner syndrome: significance of ocular features. Ophthalmology 91:916-925

Figures

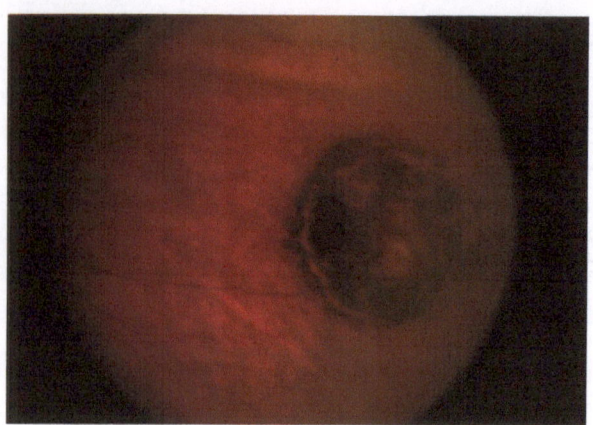

FIGURE 34-1.
These lesions are round, are well delineated, and have a halo around them. As the patient ages, depigmented lacunae are frequently seen within the body of the lesion.

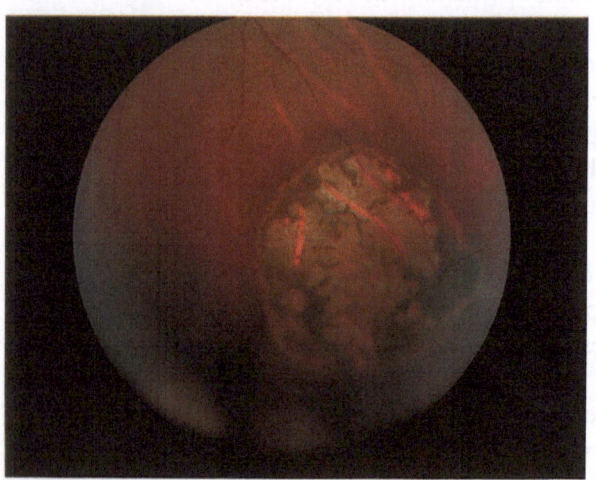

FIGURE 34-2.
Although this lesion was once total black, as the patient has grown older the depigmented lacunae have continued to coalesce. A significant amount of pigment has been lost.

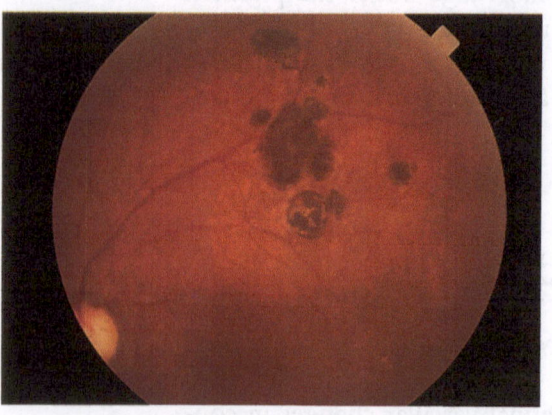

FIGURE 34-3.
Congenital grouped pigmentation of the RPE. We commonly refer to these lesions as "bear tracks."

FIGURE 34-4.
This peripheral calotte demonstrates a clinical example of congenital pigment hypertrophy, a jet black lesion.

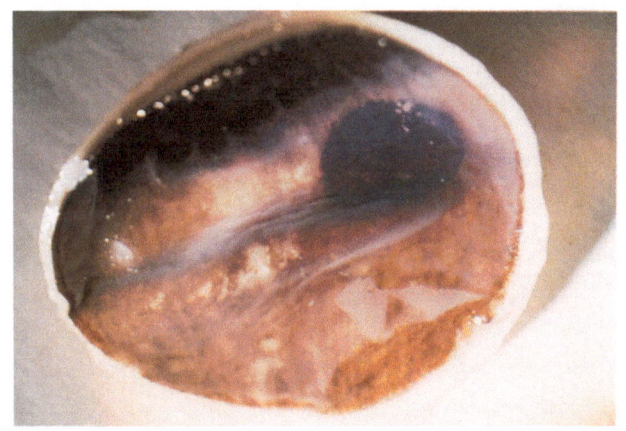

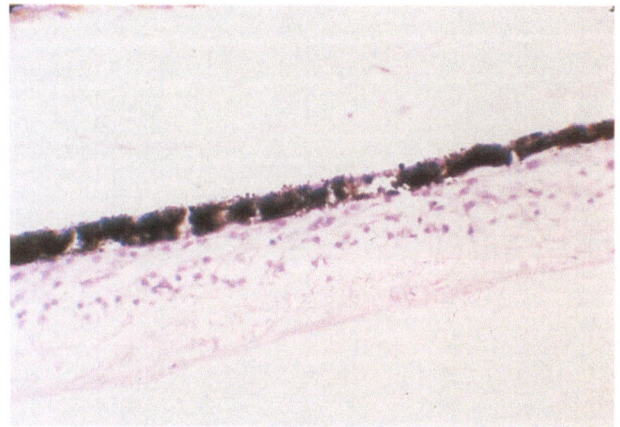

FIGURE 34-5.
Retinal pigment epithelium with enlarged pigment epithelial cells (at left). (H & E)

Chapter 35

Dominant Drusen

Drusen have been described as autosomal dominant lesions. Excrescences or nodules seen on the surface of Bruch's membrane, they may be dystrophic and familial. Characteristically, drusen located throughout the posterior pole as well as nasal to the disc for which a familial pattern can be demonstrated are commonly called dominant drusen or familial drusen. Ophthalmoscopically, they are yellow to yellow-white and are located in deep retina. They appear during the first three decades of life and are usually round. As the individual ages, the drusen may coalesce. During the fifth or sixth decade of life, a pigment epithelial detachment may occur that signals the presence of a subretinal neovascular membrane. Patients do not notice a loss of acuity until after age 40. Clinically, the number and size of the drusen increase over time.

Clinical testing reveals normal color vision. The fluorescein angiogram demonstrates window defects corresponding to the drusen present. The fluorescein usually pinpoints many more drusen than were appreciable by clinical evaluation of the fundus alone. Hyperfluorescence can be seen when a neurosensory detachment occurs. Fluorescein is indispensible for diagnosing the choroidal neovascular net that may develop in these patients. Studies show that argon laser applied to these nets is beneficial.

Electrooculography (EOG) and electroretinography (ERG) are normal. A central or paracentral defect can be seen on visual fields examination. It corresponds to the neurosensory detachment or the alteration of visual functioning cells located in the macula and paramacular zone. Typically, these patients are given an amsler grid to check their fields everyday. Color vision remains normal until the fovea is involved, signifying cone involvement. The ERG remains normal, as the ERG is a mass response. Although there have been reports of an abnormal EOG, we have not found this test to be helpful in dominant drusen patients.

Histologically, there is period acid-Schiff (PAS)-positive material (with or without calcium) deposited between the retinal pigment epithelium (RPE) and Bruch's membrane. Adjacent RPE is hyperplastic, but overlying RPE is usually atrophic.

157

Selected Reading

Deutman AF, Jansen LMAA (1970). Dominantly inherited drusen of Bruch's membrane. Br J Ophthalmol 54:373-382

Farkas TG, Krill AE, Sylvester VM, et al (1971). Familial and secondary drusen: histologic and functional correlations. Trans Am Acad Ophthalmol Otolaryngol 75:333-343

Gass JDM (1973). Drusen and disciform macular detachment and degeneration. Arch Ophthalmol 90:206-217

Figures

FIGURE 35-1.
This patient has bilateral, symmetrical drusen located between the RPE and Bruch's membrane. Some of the drusen are so large they have become confluent.

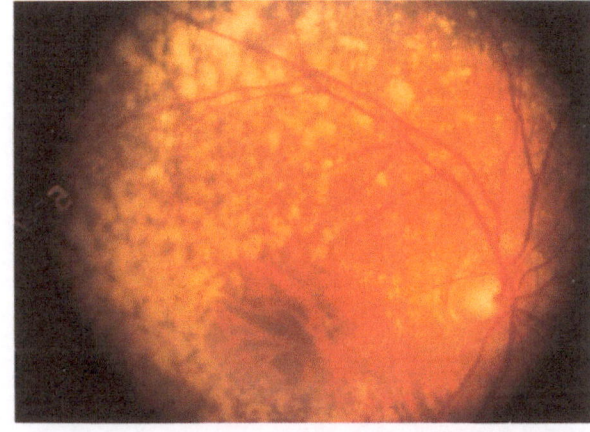

FIGURE 35-2.
Fluorescein angiography shows that the fluorescent areas coalesce; however, no neovascular net is noted.

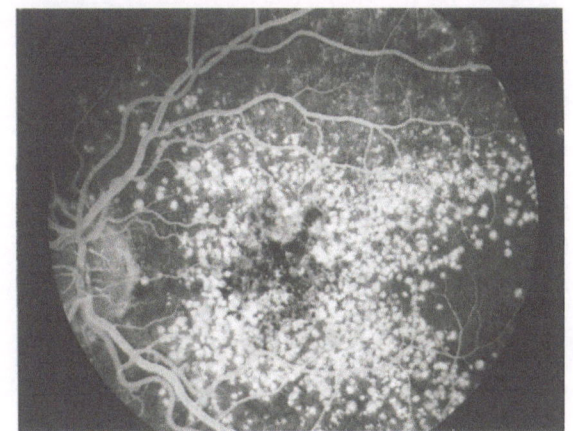

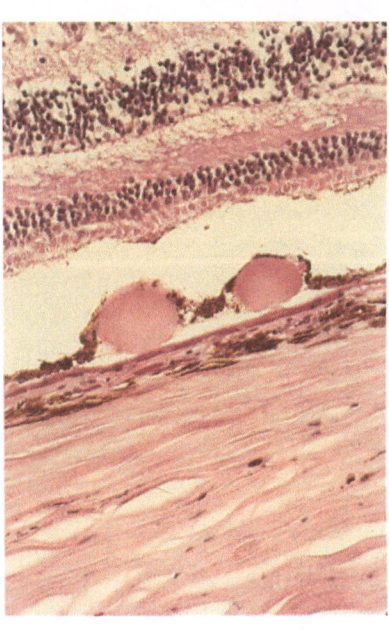

FIGURE 35-3.
Histopathology shows excrescences at the level of Bruch's membrane. (H & E)

Chapter 36

Leber's Congenital Amaurosis

Leber's congenital amaurosis has been described as an infantile form of retinitis pigmentosa (RP), although in toddlers and adults it is a separate entity. It is also called hereditary retinal blindness and Leber's congenital tapetoretinal degeneration.

These individuals have searching pendular nystagmus with the typical RP signs of optic pallor and pigmentary retinopathy. It is common to see multiple irregular white flecks located deep in the peripheral retina, which become the pigmentary spicules seen later. Visual acuity is decreased, and the pupils are poorly reactive. The refractive error is typically hyperopic. It is not unusual for these children to have renal disease, mental retardation, and neurological disturbances. The hereditary pattern is autosomal recessive. As for RP, the electroretinogram (ERG) is unrecordable, even during the neonatal period. The fluorescein angiogram is nonspecific in that it mirrors the generalized RP-like changes that are occurring. Retinal pigment epithelium atrophy is evident as hyperfluorescence, whereas blocked fluorescence is due to the retinal pigment clumping. On occasion, there is optic disc edema or even optic atrophy. Despite a severely abnormal ERG, the visual evoked potential may be preserved. Leber's congenital amaurosis remains a principal cause of congenital blindness. Associated conditions are keratoconus and cataracts.

Histopathology reveals a normal retinal pigment epithelium. The outer retinal segments seem to be shortened, however.

Selected Reading

Merin S (1991). Inherited Eye Diseases. Diagnosis and Clinical Management. New York: Marcel Dekker

Noble KC, Carr RE (1978). Lebers' congenital amaurosis: A retrospective study of 33 cases and a histopathological study of one case. Arch Ophthalmol 96:818-821

Figures

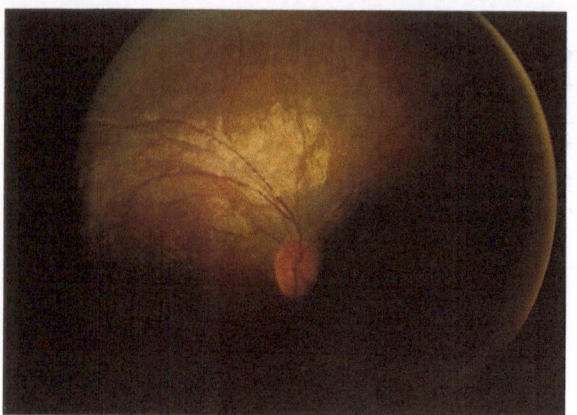

FIGURE 36-1.
This child had had poor vision and nystagmus since infancy. Note the changes in the retinal pigment epithelium. The pupils were unreactive in either eye. (Courtesy of Scott Brodie, M.D.)

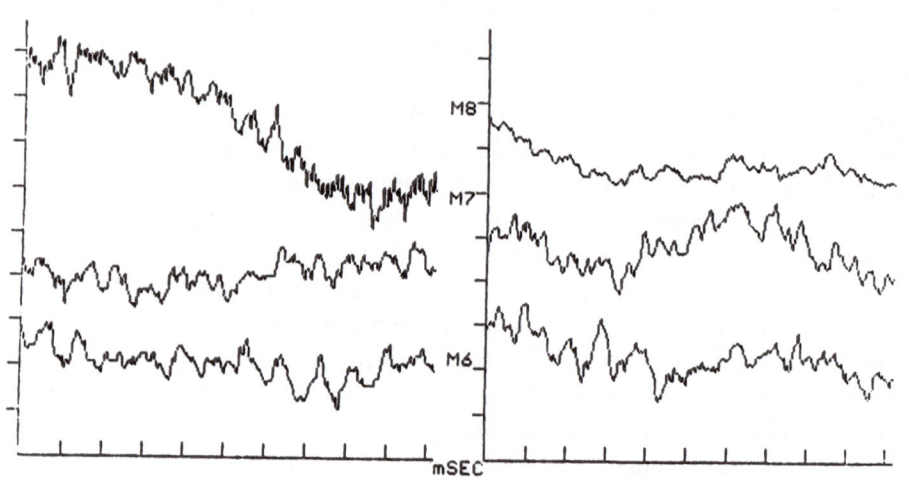

FIGURE 36-2.
Typically, the electroretinogram is nonrecordable, or flat. (Courtesy of Scott Brodie, M.D.)

Chapter 37

Retinitis Pigmentosa

Retinitis pigmentosa is one of the more common inherited retinal dystrophies. Its presenting symptoms of nyctalopia and constricted visual fields usually alerts the ophthalmologist to its diagnosis. The classic signs of the disease are "bone spicule" pigmentation (representing perivascular accumulation of the pigment epithelium melanin), thin attenuated arteries, and waxy pallor of the optic nerve. Electrophysiological testing usually reveals a nonrecordable electroretinogram (ERG) and the visual fields are either constricted or a ring scotoma is seen. Classically, the sporadic and autosomal recessive types are the more frequent forms of the disease, although X-linked and autosomal dominant forms exist. The prognosis for the recessive and X-linked groups is poor; that is, visual acuity diminishes more rapidly in these patients than in the autosomal dominant group.

Some patients have disc pallor and vessel attenuation without demonstrating the pigment dispersion or "bone-spicule" picture. The fundus usually has a slightly grayish or greenish hue; and careful observation of the periphery usually reveals minimal spicule formation. It may be seen in only one quadrant and may consist of only one or two spicules. These patients have retinitis pigmentosa sine pigmento and the electrophysiological and visual field abnormalities associated with "pigmented" retinitis pigmentosa.

In severe cases, the patients complain of night blindness during the first decade of life. Several years ago, a 3-year-old female child was seen with the complete picture of retinitis pigmentosa. Her parents had initially sought psychiatric help because the child had explosive temper tantrums when they turned off the lights in their home at night. Associated ocular findings included myopia, posterior capsular cataracts, drusen of the optic disc, and macular changes (cystoid macular edema, which causes loss of central acuity, and an epiretinal membrane). Acetazolamide (Diamox) therapy has sometimes helped to improve visual acuity in patients with cystoid macular edema.

Visual acuity can vary from 20/20 to no light perception, depending on the stage of the disease. Also varying with the stage of the disease is the visual field (constriction or ring scotomas) and the ERG. The ERG may be abnormal years before patients demonstrate any clinical signs of the disease. There is abnormal dark adaptation, and the electrooculogram is abnormal. The fluorescein angiogram depicts the status of the retinal pigment epithelium (RPE). The migrated epithelium shows hypofluorescence, and at later stages atrophy of the choriocapillaris is evident.

Histologically, the earliest changes appear to be located in the RPE and rods. With time, the rods totally degenerate, and the RPE both degenerates and proliferates. There is gliosis and loss of the inner retinal layers. The pigment tends to gravitate toward the vessels, and the retina can be seen to have pigment-laden macrophages.

Other rod-cone dystrophies in this family include sector retinitis pigmentosa, unilateral retinitis pigmentosa, inverse retinitis pigmentosa, pericentral retinitis pigmentosa, retinitis punctata albescens (not fundus albipuctata), Leber's congenital amaurosis, adult-onset retinitis pigmentosa, and pigmented paravenous chorioretinal atrophy. There are many syndromes associated with retinitis pigmentosa (see Merin and Auerbach in the Selected Reading list) and deafness has been well established as a trait that when coexisting with retinitis pigmentosa, denotes a separate family of syndromes: Usher syndrome, Bardet-Moon-Biedl syndrome, Kearns-Sayre syndrome, myotonic dystrophy, Bassen-Kornzweig syndrome, Refsum's disease, and olivopontocerebellar retinal degeneration.

Autosomal dominant retinitis pigmentosa is one of the diseases for which gene mapping has been performed. There appears to be a codon mutation that substitutes one amino acid for another. These patients have a 50% risk of having an affected child.

Selected Reading

Berson EL, Rosen JB, Simonoff EA (1979). Electroretinographic testing as an aid in detection of carriers of X-chromosome linked retinitis pigmentosa. Am J Ophthalmol 87:460-468

Boughman JA, Conneally PM, Nance WE (1980). Population genetic studies of retinitis pigmentosa. Am J Hum Genet 32:223-235

Fishman GA (1981). Color vision defects in retinitis pigmentosa. Ann Ophthalmol 13:609-618

Fishman GA, Young RSL, Vasquez V, et al (1976). Progressive human cone-rod dysfunction (dystrophy). Trans Am Acad Ophthalmol Otolaryngol 81:716-724

Heckenlively JR (1988). Retinitis Pigmentosa. Philadelphia: Lippincott

Marmor MF (1979). The electroretinogram in retinitis pigmentosa. Arch Ophthalmol 97:1300-1304

Merin S, Auerbach E (1976). Retinitis pigmentosa. Surv Ophthalmol 20:303-346

Pearlman JT, Flood TP, Seiff SR (1976). Retinitis pigmentosa without pigment. Am J Ophthalmol 81:417-419

Figures

FIGURE 37-1.
This 12-year-old female child has Lawrence-Moon-Bardet-Biedel syndrome with retinitis pigmentosa. She has extra digits on both hands. Her electroretinogram had a nonrecordable a-wave and b-wave.

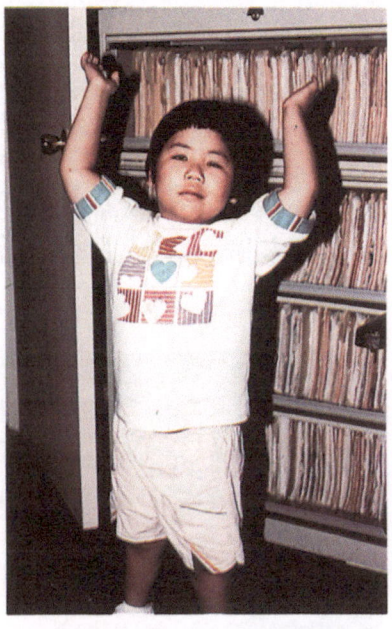

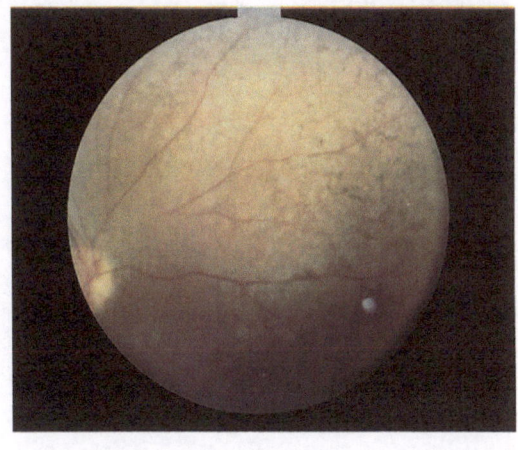

FIGURE 37-2.
Fundus of the patient in Fig. 37-1. She has the typical pigment epithelial changes called "bone spicules."

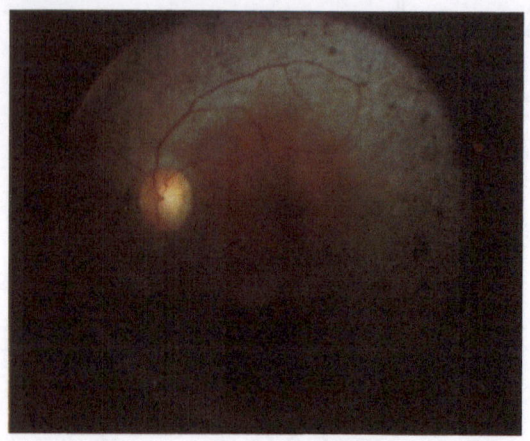

FIGURE 37-3.
This patient has attenuated retinal vessels, pigment spicules, and pallor of the disc, commonly seen with retinitis pigmentosa. Macular edema is often evident as well.

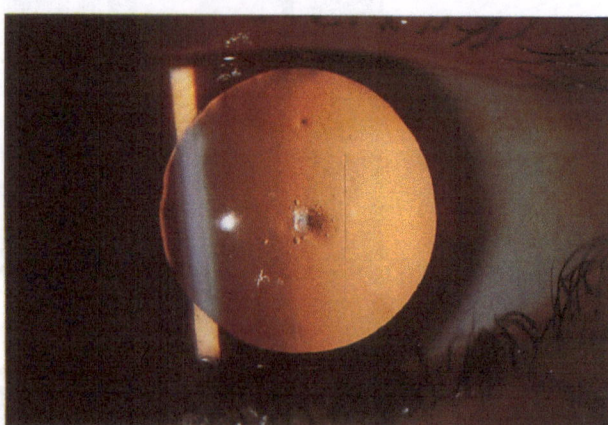

FIGURE 37-4.
Posterior subcapsular cataract in the patient in Fig. 37-3. Often the quality of vision improves after cataract surgery in these patients.

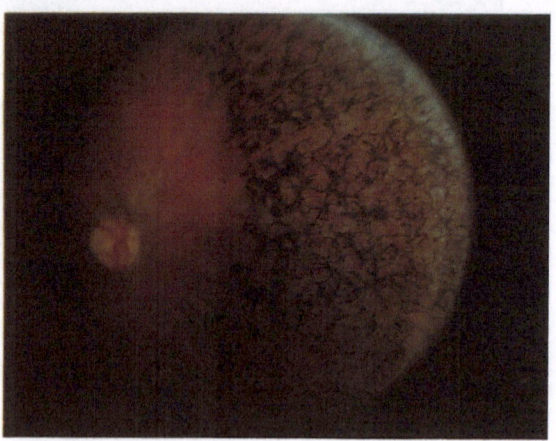

FIGURE 37-5.
Extensive bone spicules are present. This picture is distinctive, with the spicules resembling overlying, multiple, short, black threads.

FIGURE 37-6.

(A) At the age of 55, the patient noted that he had difficulty seeing at night. An ocular examination was normal. Six years later, his acuity was at the count fingers level. At age 66, now, he has attenuated vessels and optic pallor, and an island of vision remains. Francois suggested that there was a population of individuals who develop this progressive retinitis pigmentosa during their sixth decade. (B) Fluorescein angiogram demonstrates the island left after baring the choroid. An ERG was nonrecordable.

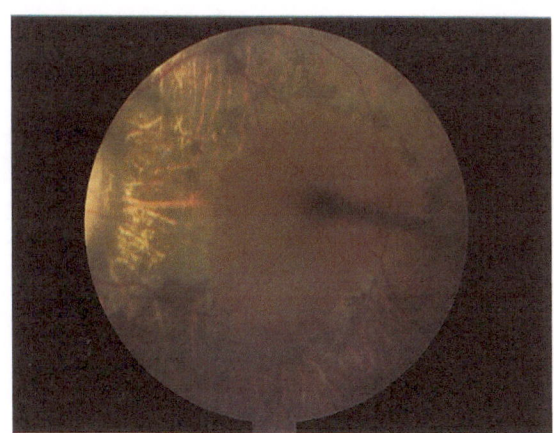

A

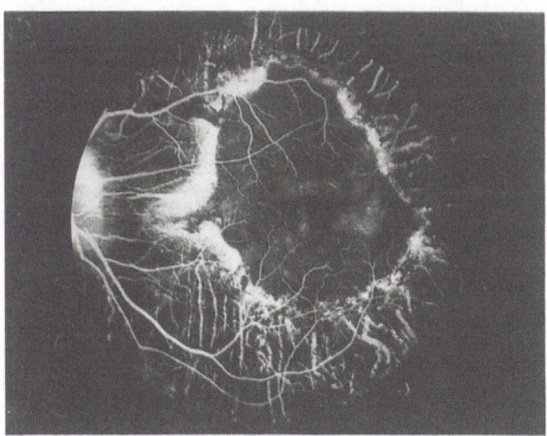

B

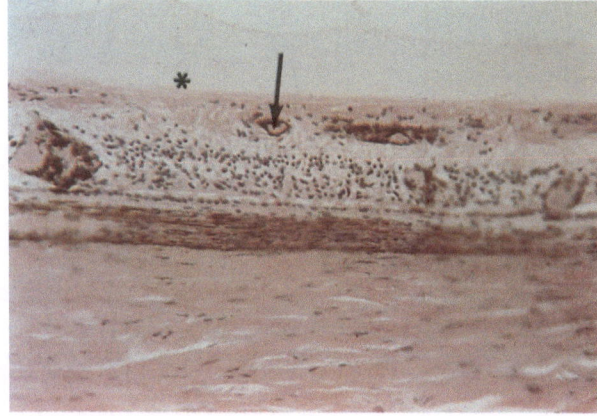

FIGURE 37-7.

Retinitis pigmentosa. Note the atrophy of the outer retina, that is, a loss of photoreceptors and outer nuclear layers. There is pigment migration into the retina and around the vessels. (arrow) A preretinal glial membrane is present. (*) (H & E)

Chapter 38

Pigmented Paravenous Retinochoroidal Atrophy

Pigmented paravenous retinochoroidal atrophy appears much like retinitis pigmentosa to the uninitiated. Indeed there are many patients who have this disorder and spend a great deal of their life expecting to become blind. Funduscopically, these patients demonstrate retinal pigment spicules clustered around the retinal veins. Clinically, some have a mild nyctalopia and mild decrease in acuity; however, the optic atrophy, arteriolar narrowing, and progression of retinitis pigmentosa are not present. Electrophysiologically, we have seen normal photopic and scotopic electroretinograms. The fluorescein angiogram demonstrates a hypofluorescence around the veins that corresponds to the perivascular location of the spicules. There is also a decrease in the retinal pigment epithelium around the fovea. Macular fields show decreased perifoveal values, consistent with the hypopigmented perifoveal region. It seems that this disorder remains stable, without progression, over several years. It is unclear whether the entity is congenital or acquired from another illness. Genetic studies suggest that inheritance is sporadic.

Selected Reading

Chisolm IA, Dudgeon J (1973). Pigmented paravenous retino-choroidal atrophy: helicoid retino-choroidal atrophy. Br J Ophthalmol 57:584-587

Hirose T, Miyake Y (1979). Pigmentary paravenous chorioretinal degeneration: fundus appearance and retinal functions. Ann Ophthalmol 11:709-718

Noble RG, Carr RE (1983). Pigmented paravenous chorioretinal atrophy. Am J Ophthalmol 96:338-344

Small KW, Anderson Jr WB (1991). Pigmented paravenous retinochoroidal atrophy: discordant expression in monozygotic twins. Arch Ophthalmol 109:1408-1410

Figures

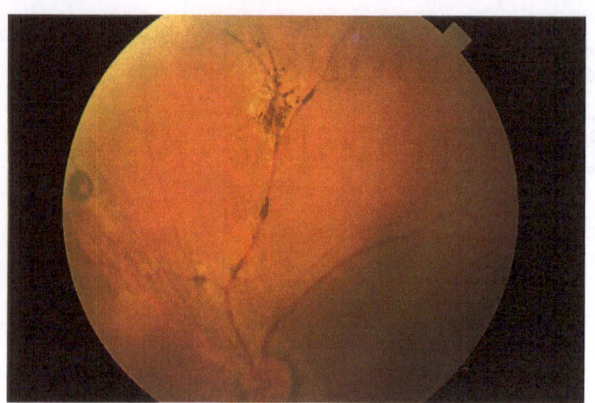

FIGURE 38-1.
This patient was seen for a second opinion because an ophthalmologist told her that she had retinitis pigmentosa. Patients with pigmented paravenous retinochoroidal atrophy have pigment migration solely to the area around the retinal veins.

Chapter 39

Stargardt's Disease

Stargardt's disease is an autosomal recessive condition in which the retina displays characteristic yellow flecks often associated with macular degeneration. The degeneration appears similar to that seen with fundus flavimaculatus. It is debated, however, whether these two entities are distinct or represent two points on the spectrum of a single disease. There are as many investigators who "split" them as there are who "lump" them. Herein, they are considered to be a single entity.

Typically, the patients present as young adults with blurred vision. The macular region has an irregularity of the pigment epithelium. Other patients show a beaten-bronze appearance. The classic picture is one of multiple white flecks in the posterior pole extending both nasally to the disc and outside the arcades. These flecks have been called "pisciform" (fish-like) in appearance. When there is frank atrophy of the macula, optic atrophy may be seen. This autosomal recessive disorder is progressive and leaves the patient with severe visual loss in cases where macular atrophy ensues.

As with some other diseases, such as congenital stationary night blindness, retinitis pigmentosa, and gyrate atrophy, the refraction is myopic in fundus flavimaculatus. There are no typical color vision abnormalities. Other entities that involve the photoreceptors have color vision abnormalities, whereas disorders involving the pigment epithelium have normal color vision. At worst, the visual fields demonstrate constriction. If the macula is severely affected, the fields have a central scotoma. Fluorescein angiography is useful in cases of fundus flavimaculatus. The macula can demonstrate a bull's eye. Patches of hypofluorescence are due to the flecks. The choroidal picture is almost pathognomonic. Despite macular atrophy, the choroid appears to be silent; it is not visualized. Electroretinography (ERG) evaluation is typically normal or slightly reduced in the photopic mode. In the scotopic mode the ERG is normal. The electrooculogram is abnormal in most cases.

Selected Reading

Eagle RC, Lucier AC, Bernardino VB, et al (1980). Retinal pigment epithelial abnormalities in fundus flavimaculatus: a light and electron microscopic study. Ophthalmology 87:1189-1200

Fishman GA (1976). Fundus flavimaculatus: a clinical classification. Arch Ophthalmol 94:2061-2067

Noble KG, Carr RE (1979). Stargardt's disease and fundus flavimaculatus. Arch Ophthalmol 97:1281-1285

Stargardt K (1909). Über familiare, progressive Degeneration in der Makulagegend des Auges. Graefes Arch Ophthalmol 71:534-550

Figures

FIGURE 39-1.
This young boy noted a loss of central vision. On examination acuity was 20/100, and there were yellow pigment flecks in the macula. The flecks surround the macula and are located within the retinal pigment epithelium.

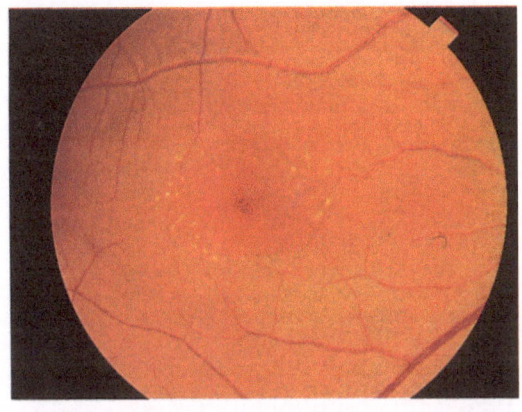

FIGURE 39-2.
This woman presented with a bull's-eye pattern of retinal pigment atrophy.

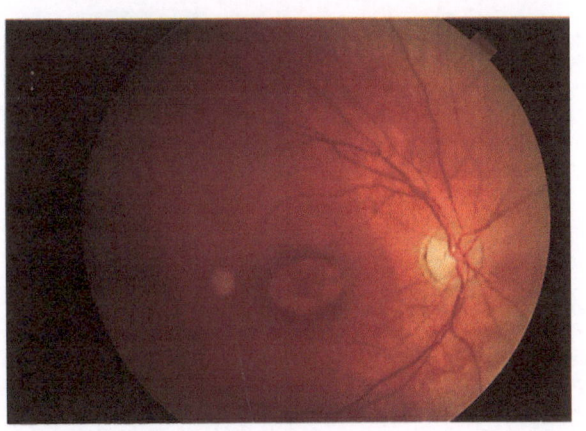

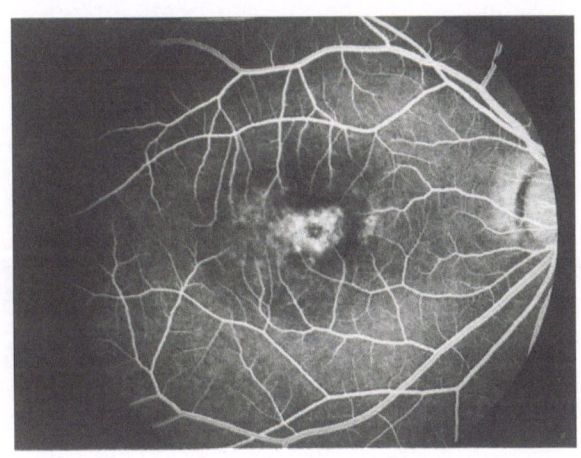

FIGURE 39-3.
Fluorescein angiogram depicting the RPE pigment abnormalities seen around the fovea.

Section 8

Choroid

Chapter 40

Central Areolar Choroidal Dystrophy

Central areolar choroidal dystrophy presents with an abnormality in the patient's central acuity. Usually the defect is mild, but it may progress to legal blindness. In its early stages the macular region has a pigment epithelial irregularity, and as the disease progresses, an oval or round region around the fovea becomes apparent. The pigment epithelium and choriocapillaris become atrophic, baring the larger choroidal vasculature. Some of the pigment epithelium may clump within this central area.

The hereditary pattern is autosomal dominant. There is characteristically a slow progression that begins during the patient's early thirties. Visual field testing elucidates a central scotoma. The color vision is abnormal, and the electroretinogram is reduced. Generally the electrooculogram is normal. The fluorescein angiogram relects the state of both the pigment epithelial and choriocapillaris integrity. A transmission defect is noted during the early stages.

Selected Reading

Ashton N (1953). Central areolar choroidal sclerosis: a histopathological study. Br J Ophthalmol 37:140-147

Noble KG (1977). Central areolar choroidal dystrophy. Am J Ophthalmol 84:310-318

Sorsby A, Crick RP (1953). Central areolar choroidal sclerosis. Br J Ophthalmol 37:129-139

Figures

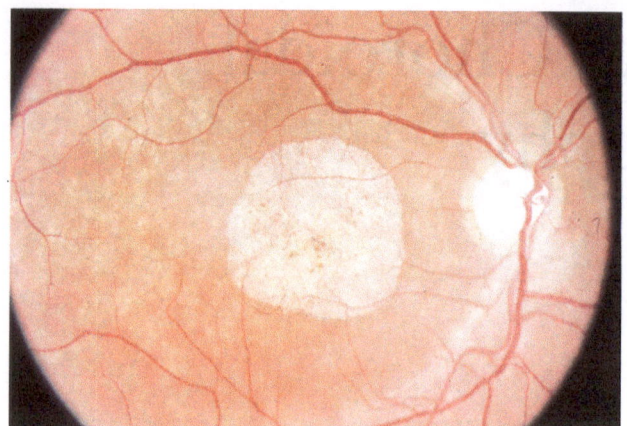

FIGURE 40-1.
Loss of central visual acuity was noted in this patient; acuity is 20/200. There is atrophy of the RPE, especially around the fovea, and generalized RPE atrophy throughout the retina.

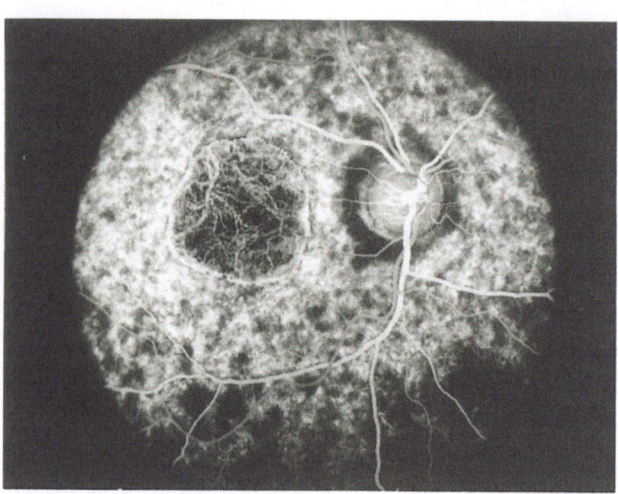

FIGURE 40-2.
Fluorescein angiogram showing a plethora of transmission defects. Some of the larger choroidal vessels are visible in the inferior portion of the photograph. This picture is indicative of a patient with long-standing disease.

Chapter 41

Choroideremia

Patients (primarily men) with choroideremia complain of an abnormality of their visual fields, a loss of visual acuity, and nyctalopia. This bilaterally progressive condition is rarely seen during childhood. There are several stages to the disease. During the early period, examination of the fundus reveals a midperipheral "salt and pepper" picture. Although the macula is spared, the choriocapillaris and choroidal vasculature atrophy. During the late stages of the disease, visual acuity is diminished. The vessels are attenuated, and the macula becomes affected. The choroid is generally atrophied to varying degrees throughout the fundus.

Genetically, choroideremia is inherited as an X-linked recessive condition. It has been called progressive tapetochoroidal dystrophy or diffuse total choroidal vascular atrophy of X-linked inheritance. Fluorescein angiography demonstrates window defects with diffuse hyperfluorescence. As the disease progresses areas of hypofluoresecence appear that reflect choroidal atrophy. The visual fields demonstrate constriction. Color vision can be variably affected, often exhibiting tritanopia. The electroretinogram is unrecordable during the late stages, and the electrooculogram is abnormal. Female carriers of the disease have a brown fundus with pigment stippling and peripapillary atrophy of the retinal pigment epithelium.

Histologically, the choroid disappears, and there is atrophy of the outer retinal layers.

Selected Reading

Ayazi S (1981). Choroideremia, obesity, and congenital deafness. Am J Ophthalmol 92:63-69

Hayasaka S, Shoji K, Kanno CL, et al (1985). Differential diagnosis of diffuse choroidal atrophies: diffuse choriocapillaris atrophy, choroideremia, and gyrate atrophy of the choroid and retina. Retina 5:30-37

Rodrigues MM, Ballintine EJ, Wiggert BN, et al (1984). Choroideremia: a clinical, electron microscopic, and biochemical report. Ophthalmology 91:873-883

Rubin ML, Fishman RS, McKay RA (1966). Choroideremia: study of a family and literature review. Arch Ophthalmol 76:563-574

Figures

FIGURE 41-1.
Choroideremia manifests during childhood and continues to progress throughout the adult years. The choroid becomes atrophic,as do, secondarily, the overlying outer layers of the retina. As can be seen in this 45-year-old patient, most of the fundus becomes yellow-white.

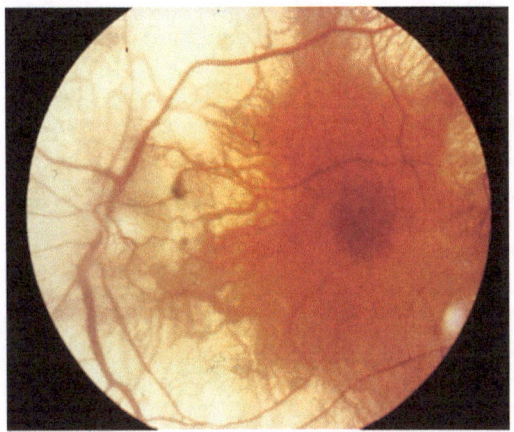

Chapter 42

Gyrate Atrophy

Patients with gyrate atrophy often complain of poor night vision. Characteristically, they are myopic. Clinically, the retina exhibits atrophic scalloped lesions in the midperiphery. The normal retina that lies between the lesions has hyperpigmented edges. Biochemically, there is a deficiency of ornithine aminotransferase. The condition affects not only the eyes but the muscular system, brain, and hair. Blood plasma levels of ornithine are greatly elevated. Cataracts (posterior subcapsular) are seen at a late stage, as are disc pallor, vessel attenuation, and myopia.

The condition is inherited as autosomal recessive and is slowly progressive. Acuity may be normal, but it eventually decreases to 20/200 or worse. The fluorescein angiogram demonstrates loss of the choriocapillaris and retinal pigment epithelium. The region between lesions is normal, although even clinically normal tissue may demonstrate increased visibility of the larger choroidal vessels. The dark-adaptation curve shows high thresholds. The visual fields demonstrate scotomas, and color vision is normal. Electrophysiologically, the electroretinogram (ERG) shows an abnormal scotopic pattern that converts to an absent ERG as the disease progresses. The electrooculogram is abnormal.

Some patients respond to pyridoxine (vitamin B6) with a reduction of plasma ornithine levels (a few patients), whereas most other patients show no response. The clinical response to pyridoxine is seen in patients with both genetic forms of the disease.

Selected Reading

Kaiser-Kupfer MI, Caruso RC, Valle D (1991). Gyrate atrophy of the choroid and retina: long-term reduction of ornithine slows retinal degeneration. Arch Ophthalmol 109:1539-1548

Kaiser-Kupfer MI, Valle D, Del Valle LA (1978). A specific enzyme defect in gyrate atrophy. Am J Ophthalmol 85:200-204

Simell O, Takki K (1973). Raised plasma ornithine and gyrate atrophy of the choroid and retina. Lancet 1:1031-1033

Takki KK, Milton RC (1981). The natural history of gyrate atrophy of the choroid and retina. Ophthalmology 88:292-301

Figures

FIGURE 42-1.
Diffuse total choroidal vascular atrophy or gyrate atrophy of the choroid. The patient presented with slowly decreasing vision and nyctalopia. Atrophic, scalloped chorioretinal patches of atrophy started in the periphery and traveled toward the posterior pole.

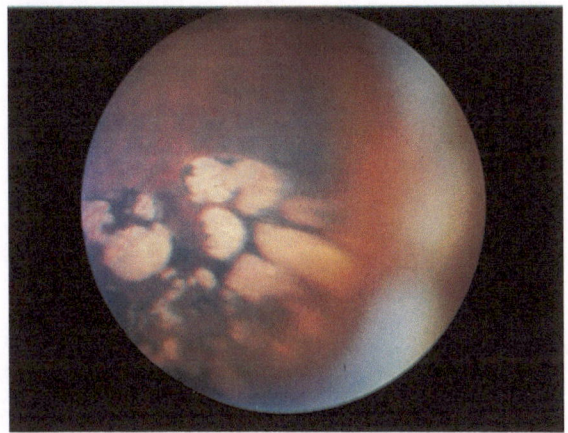

Section 9

Phakomatoses

Chapter 43

Ataxia-Telangiectasia

Louis-Bar syndrome, or ataxia-telangiectasia, is considered by most investigators to be one of the phakomatoses. It begins during childhood, typically with cerebellar ataxia, multiple pulmonary infections, and chronic dry skin. The patients have lymphocytic abnormalities, which may be the etiology for the infections as well as the skin changes. These patients have nystagmus and characteristic conjunctival dilated and telangiectatic vessels. In the retina, microaneurysms and vessel tortuosity have been described. It is inherited in an autosomal recessive pattern.

Selected Reading

Boder E, Sedgwick RP (1958). Ataxia-telangiectasia: a familial syndrome of progressive cerebellar ataxia, oculocutaneous telangiectasia and frequent pulmonary infection. Pediatrics 21:526-554

Louis-Bar D (1941). Sur un syndrome progressif comprenant des telangiectasis capillaires cutanees et conjunctivales symetriques a disposition navoide et des troubles cerebelleux. Confin Neurol 4:32-50

Figures

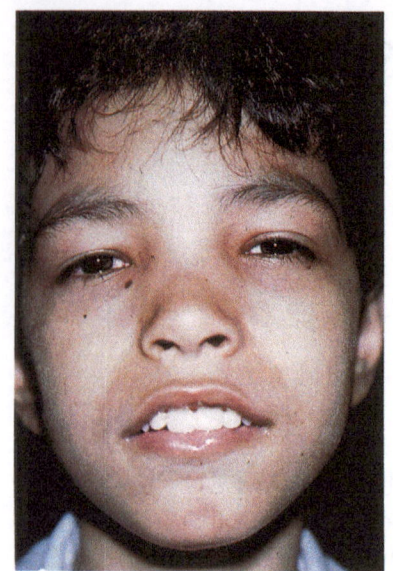

A

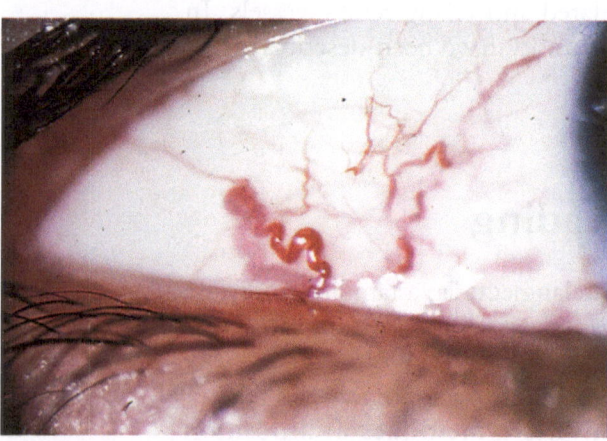

B

FIGURE 43-1.
(A) This child is so ataxic he is unable to walk. The ataxia began when he was 7 years of age, and he is currently 12. (B) Telangiectatic conjunctival vessels suggest the diagnosis of Louis-Bar syndrome.

Chapter 44

Neurofibromatosis

Neurofibromatosis encompasses a vast array of ophthalmic manifestations. It is probably one of the most common autosomal dominant diseases and is one of the phakomatoses. The classic form of neurofibromatosis, von Recklinghausen's disease, usually involves the eye in some manner.

Neurofibromas can be seen on the eyelids and can cause extensive distortion of the lids, leading to effective patching of the individual's eye as well as a ptosis. The cornea has thickened nerves. Glaucoma may also be present secondary to an anomaly of the angle. Typically, iris hamartomas, or Lisch nodules, can be seen. The Lisch nodules are melanocytic nevi. Choroidal nevi appear to be more frequent and may produce the high number of malignant melanomas in this patient population. These nevi, scattered throughout the choroid, are composed of Schwann cells associated with an increased number of densely packed cells with small nuclei. Retinal lesions are unusual. Gliomas of the optic nerve have also been associated with neurofibromatosis. These patients have visual loss, optic nerve head pallor, proptosis, and an abnormal visual field.

Although the disease is present in 1 of every 3000 neonates, it expresses itself at different times. Involvement may become evident during infancy, childhood, or even adulthood.

Selected Reading

Croxatto JO, Charles DE, Malbran E (1981). Neurofibromatosis associated with nevus of Ota and choroidal melanoma. Am J Ophthalmol 92:578-580

Font RL, Ferry AP (1972). The phakomatoses. Int Ophthalmol Clin 12(1):1-50

Lewis RA, Riccardi VM (1981). von Recklinghausen neurofibromatosis: incidence of iris hamartomata. Ophthalmology 88:348-354

Perry HD, Font RL (1982). Iris nodules in von Recklinghausen's neurofibromatosis: electron-microscopic confirmation of their melanocytic origin. Arch Ophthalmol 100:1635-1640

Wolter JR (1966). Corneal involvement in choroidal neurofibromatosis. J Pediatr Ophthalmol 3(2):19-24

Figures

FIGURE 44-1.
Note the cafe au lait spots typically on the arm. They are typically seen in patients with neurofibromatosis.

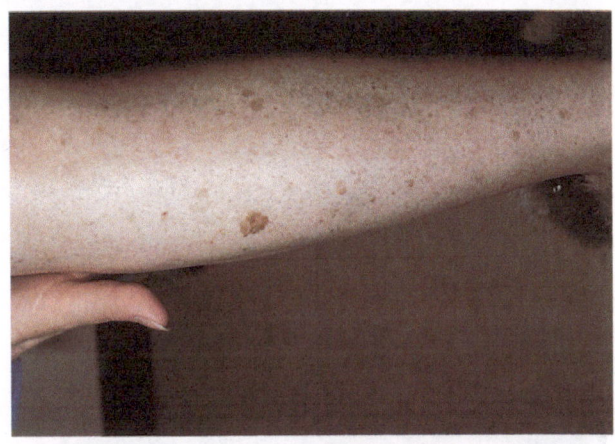

FIGURE 44-2.
Cornea may demonstrate thickened nerves.

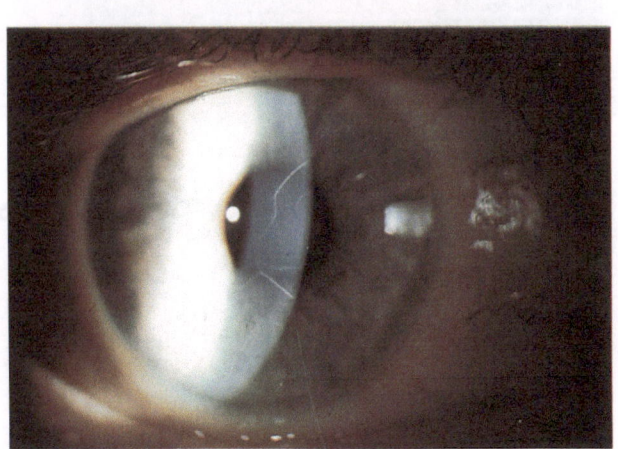

FIGURE 44-3.
(A) The optic nerve may have pallor. A computed tomography (CT) scan should be performed.

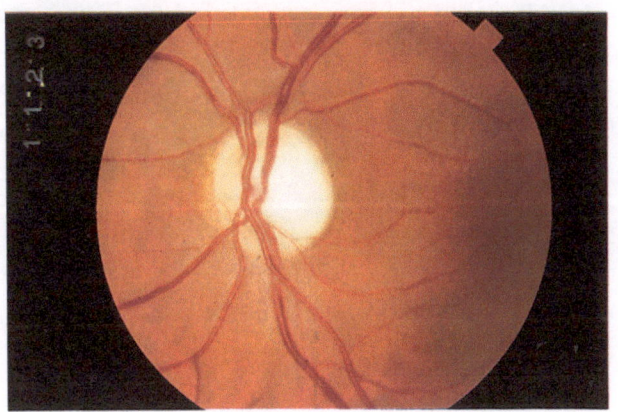

A

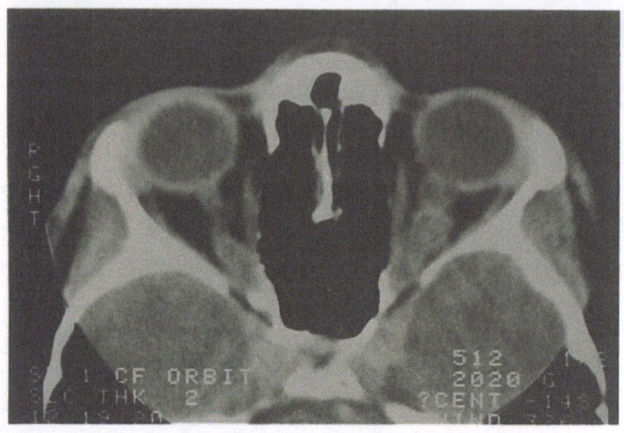

B

FIGURE 44-3. *Continued*
(B) CT scan demonstrates an enlarged optic nerve consistent with the diagnosis of optic nerve glioma.

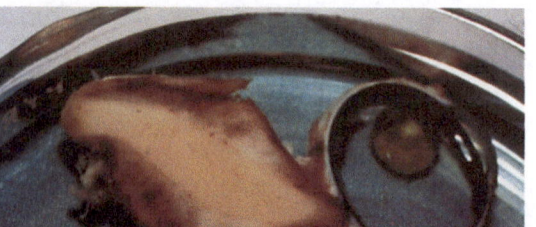

A

FIGURE 44-4.
(A) The globe was removed, and the optic nerve (ON) can be seen. (B) Histopathologically, the tumor merges into normal nerve tissue. Some of the nerve fiber bundles are enlarged owing to infiltration with glial cells. (arrow) (H & E)

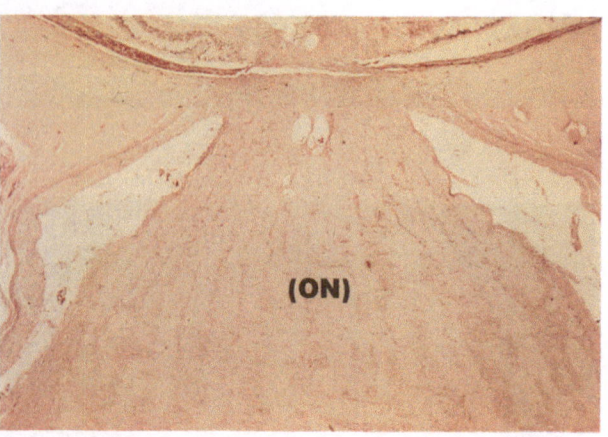

B

Chapter 45

Sturge-Weber Syndrome

Sturge-Weber syndrome, also called encephalotrigeminal angiomatosis, does not have a well delineated hereditary pattern. It is a congenital syndrome that usually has a port wine stain (nevus flammeus) with ipsilateral intracranial hemangioma, ipsilateral choroidal hemangioma, and glaucoma.

Histologically, the skin lesion is composed of proliferating, dilated, telangiectatic blood vessels within the dermis. This nevus flammeus follows the distribution of the first and second division of the fifth cranial nerve.

A racemose malformation can be seen within the cranial cavity, usually in the meninges overlying the occipital lobes. The cortex calcifies in a characteristic "railroad ties" configuration. Epilepsy is noted in more than 50% of cases.

The hemangioma is present diffusely in the choroid. The associated glaucoma is often difficult to treat. It is interesting to note that cavernous hemangiomas not associated with Sturge-Weber exist as isolated, localized choroidal lesions. Histologically, the hemangioma have dilated vascular channels. The overlying pigment epithelium displays atrophy an in some cases, metaplasia.

Suggested Reading

Atmaca LS, Kanpolat A (1983). Diagnosis and treatment of cavernous hemangiomas of the choroid and retina. Ann Ophthalmol 15:210-212

Jones IS, Cleasby GW (1959). Hemangioma of the choroid: a clinicopathologic analysis. Am J Ophthalmol 48:612-628

Stokes JJ (1957). The ocular manifestations of the Sturge-Weber syndrome. South Med J 50:82-89

Witschel H, Font RL (1976). Hemangioma of the choroid: a clinicopathologic study of 71 cases and a review of the literature. Surv Ophthalmol 20:415-431

Figures

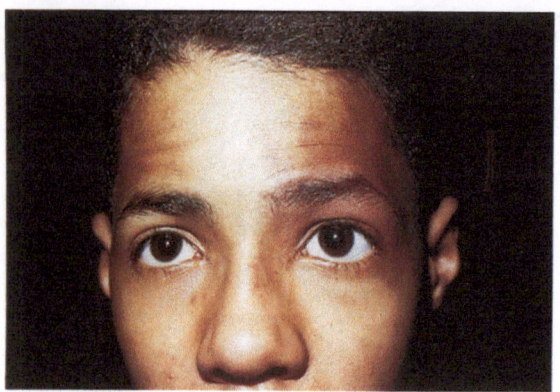

FIGURE 45-1.
Port-wine stain (nevus flammeus) in this young man with meningocutaneous angiomatosis, or Sturge-Weber syndrome.

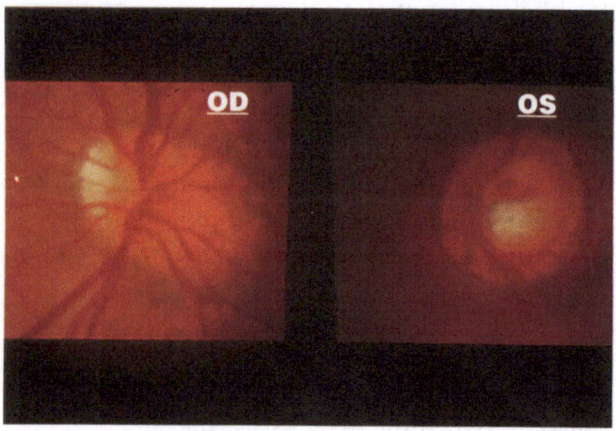

FIGURE 45-2.
Optic cup/disc ratio in the right eye is normal. (OD) The cup/disc ratio in the left eye is increased owing to the congenital glaucoma present. (OS)

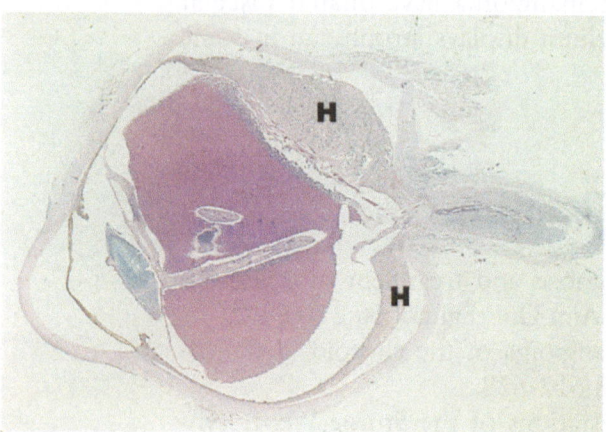

FIGURE 45-3.
Photomicrograph of an enucleated eye showing an extensive choroidal hemangioma (H) extending from ora to ora. Note the total retinal detachment. (Luxol fast blue)

FIGURE 45-4.
High-power photomicrograph depicting an extensive choroidal hemangioma. There is a serous detachment and atrophy of the overlying retina. (H & E)

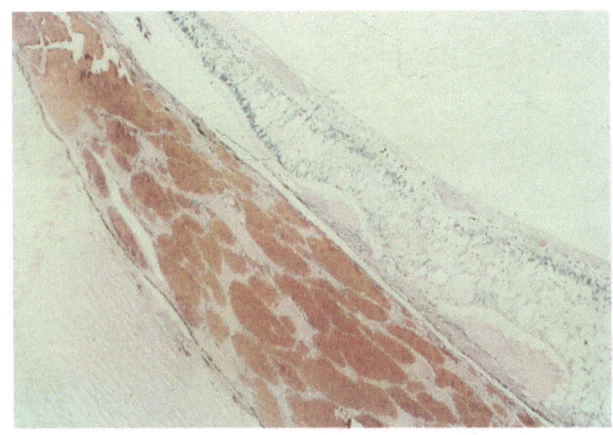

FIGURE 45-5.
Clinical photograph of a localized juxtapapillary choroidal hemangioma not associated with Sturge-Weber syndrome. Typically, these hemangiomas are well circumscribed and located in the posterior pole. (Courtesy of Joseph B. Walsh, M.D.)

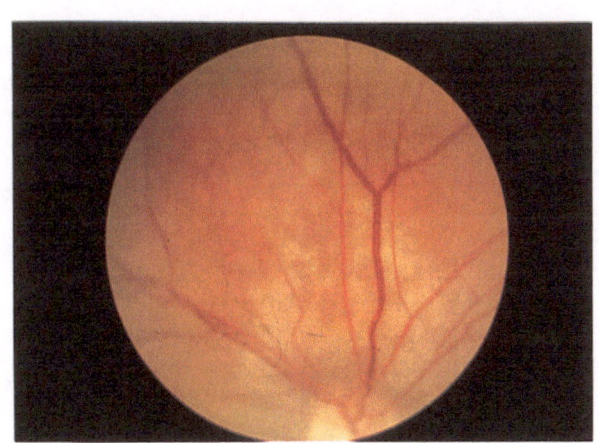

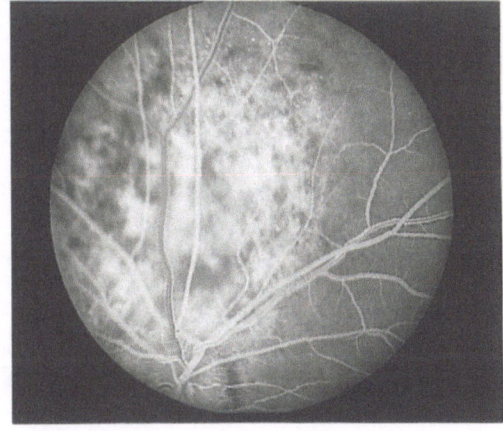

FIGURE 45-6.
Fluorescein angiogram showing the lesion to be localized just above the optic disc. (Courtesy of Joseph B. Walsh, M.D.)

Chapter 46

Cavernous Hemangioma

Gass described several patients with a cavernous hemangioma and suggested that it was part of a larger syndrome that involved the skin and brain. The disorder is inherited as an autosomal dominant condition.

Characteristically, the lesion resembles a cluster of red grapes fed by the venous system. Each grape is an aneurysm that permits separation of the erythrocytes and plasma. Thus a water mark is seen within each globule. On fluorescein angiography the lesion is seen to fill from above, and an plasma-erythrocyte interface is seen. If the grape cluster lesion extends into the macula, vision may be compromised. On occasion the lesions bleed, causing a vitreous hemorrhage. Later, they may develop a fibrotic appearance.

Photocoagulation is fraught with danger, as the aneurysm is a thin-walled venule. The vessels can easily leak if treated directly with intense therapy.

Histologically, the cavernous hemangioma is composed of endothelially lined spaces that cause an elevation of the choroid.

Selected Reading

Gass JDM (1971). Cavernous hemangioma of the retina: a neuro-oculo-cutaneous syndrome. Am J Ophthalmol 71:799-814

Lewis RA, Cohen MH, Wise GN (1975). Cavernous hemangioma of the retina and optic disc: a report of three cases and a review of the literature. Br J Ophthalmol 59:422-434

Figures

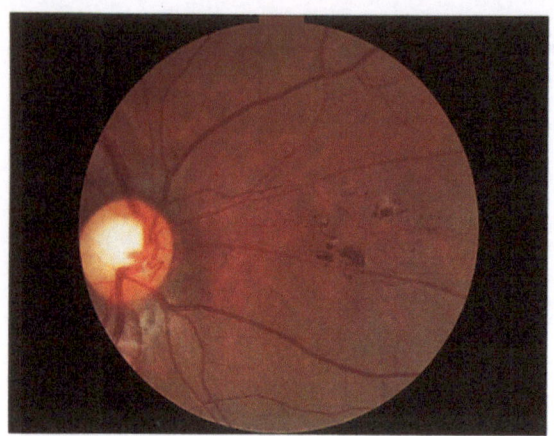

FIGURE 46-1.
Collection of grape-like abnormal vessels in the retina.

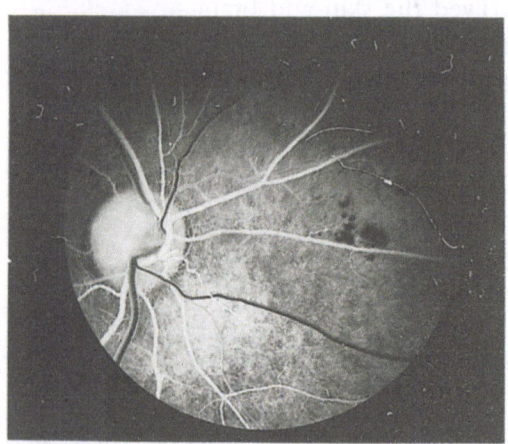

FIGURE 46-2.
In this early fluorescein angiogram, we can see that there is a delay in the filling of these lesions.

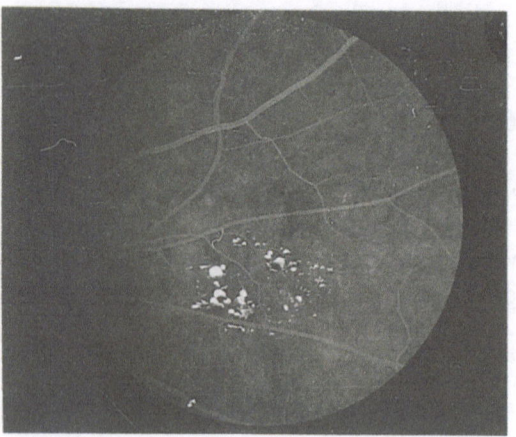

FIGURE 46-3.
Late angiogram demonstrates retention of the dye 10 minutes after the fluorescein was injected.

FIGURE 46-4.
As the hemangioma ages, it can undergo fibrosis, as seen in this example. (Courtesy of Joseph B. Walsh, M.D.)

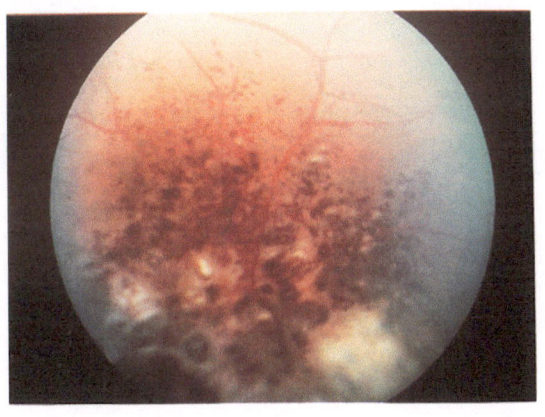

Chapter 47

Tuberous Sclerosis

Bourneville's disease was the eponym given the entity tuberous sclerosis. This condition affects the brain, skin, and eyes with hamartomatous tumors [A hamartoma is anomalous proliferation of tissue(s) usually found at that location.] It is inherited as an autosomal dominant disorder as are most of the phakomatoses. The incidence can be as high as 1 per 300 in mentally retarded populations.

The original description of tuberous sclerosis included epilepsy, mental retardation, and adenoma sebaceum. To this picture have been added astrocytic hamartomas of the optic nerve and retina. The skin lesion, a reddish rash seen on the face, is common in these patients. It appears by the end of the first decade and grows with time. There may also be hypopigmented skin macules, which comprise the ash-leaf sign.

Retinal hamartomas are seen in more than 50% of cases. The lesions may be flat and noncalcified or mulberry and calcified. A third type, a combination of the other two, has been described as well. A large percentage of these hamartomas occur near the optic nerve or overlie it. An eye can have either type of hamartoma or a combination of them. Abnormalities of pigmentation may result in both hyper- and hypopigmented areas. Vitreous hemorrhage arising from these tumors or associated neovascularization have been reported by various investigators.

Fluorescein angiography demonstrates a plethora of capillary channels in the astrocytic hamartomas of tuberous sclerosis. Electrophysiological studies are typically normal. Histologically the tumors are located in the superficial layers of the retina and composed of proliferative astroglia.

Selected Reading

Atkinson A, Sanders MD, Wong V (1973). Vitreous hemorrhage in tuberous sclerosis: report of two cases. Br J Ophthalmol 57:773-779

De Juan Jr E, Green WR, Gupta PK, Baranano EC (1984). Vitreous seeding by retinal astrocytic hamartoma in a patient with tuberous sclerosis. Retina 4:100-102

Guttman I, Dunn D, Behrens M, et al (1982). Hypopigmented iris spot: an early sign of tuberous sclerosis. Ophthalmology 89:1155-1159

Williams R, Taylor D (1985). Tuberous sclerosis. Surv Ophthalmol 30:143-154

Figures

FIGURE 47-1.
Tuberous sclerosis. There is an astrocytic lesion on the optic nerve head, and the lesion is globular, well defined, and elevated. This child had seizures and mental retardation.

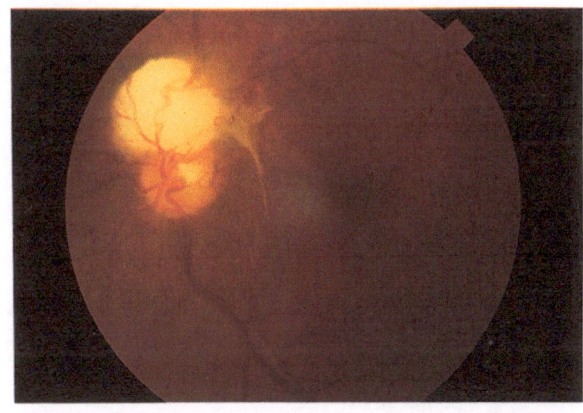

FIGURE 47-2.
Calcified retinal astrocytic hamartoma. Retinal hamartomas show less tendency to undergo calcification, and they rarely grow.

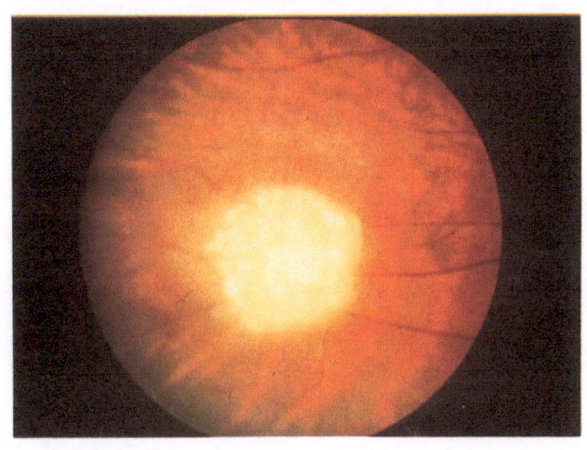

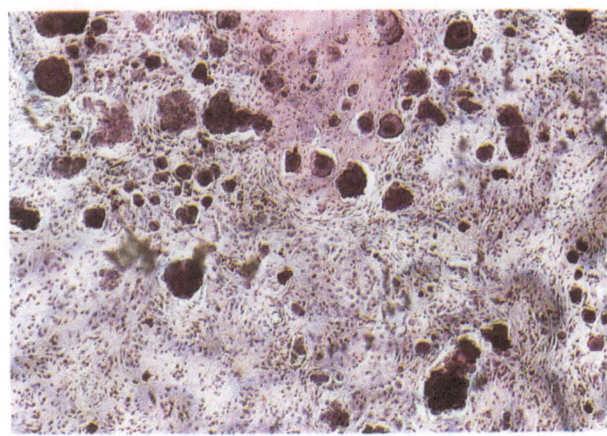

FIGURE 47-3.
This retinal astrocystic hamartoma was found at autopsy. Note the calcifications present within the tumor. (H & E)

Figures

Chapter 48

Von Hippel-Lindau Disease

The angiomas of von Hippel-Lindau disease can affect many organ systems and sometimes undergo malignant transformation. The disease, an autosomal dominant with incomplete penetrance, affects the brain, eye, spinal cord, lungs, adrenals, and liver. Certainly its most characteristic features are angiomas of the retina and brain. The disease occurs more often than tuberous sclerosis but less often than neurofibromatosis.

The retina contains a yellow-red mass, or angioma, in the periphery with arteriole or venous feeder vessels. These angiomas may be small or large. There may be more than one angioma per eye, and in more than 50% of patients they appear bilaterally. Although some angiomas remain stable over many years, others cause a significant amount of damage. Secondary leakage from the angiomas can cause retinal edema, hard exudate formation (especially in the macula), serous detachment of the retina, and either a subretinal or a vitreous hemorrhage.

The central nervous system can harbor hemangiomas or hemangioblastomas of the cerebellum. Other benign or malignant lesions may also occur. Therapy can be accomplished with xenon arc, argon laser, or cryoretinopexy of the lesion; it is suggested that the burns be large, of long duration, and of low intensity. Certain tumors can also be treated by eye wall resection. If sucessfully treated, the angiomas demonstrate occlusion of the vascular malformation and subsequent involution.

Selected Reading

Goldberg MF (1977). Clinicopathological correlation of von Hippel angiomas after xenon arc and laser photocoagulation. In GA Peyman, DJ Apple, DR Sanders (eds): Intraocular Tumors. Norwalk, CT: Appleton-Century-Crofts

Hardwig P, Robertson DM (1984). Von Hippel-Lindau disease: a familial, often lethal, multi-system phakomatosis. Ophthalmology 91:263-270

Mottow-Lippa L, Tso MOM, Peyman GA, Chejfec G (1983). von Hippel angiomatosis: a light, electron microscopic, and immunoperoxidase characterization. Ophthalmology 90:848-855

Figures

FIGURE 48-1.
Note the capillary hemangioma located superotemporal to the optic nerve. The retinal component, a capillary hemangioma of the retina, was initially described by von Hippel and so the condition was called von Hippel's disease. This patient also had a spinal cord hemangioma. Her sister had a capillary hemangioma that bled and caused a massive vitreous hemorrhage.

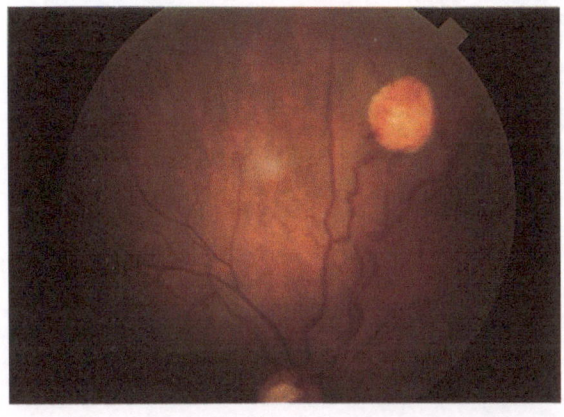

FIGURE 48-2.
Close-up view of the hemangioma shows that it is elevated and highly vascular.

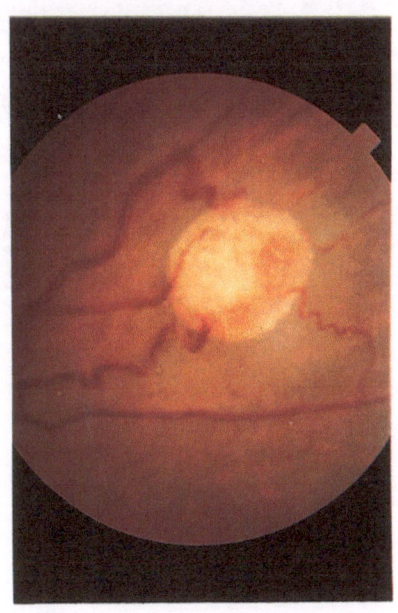

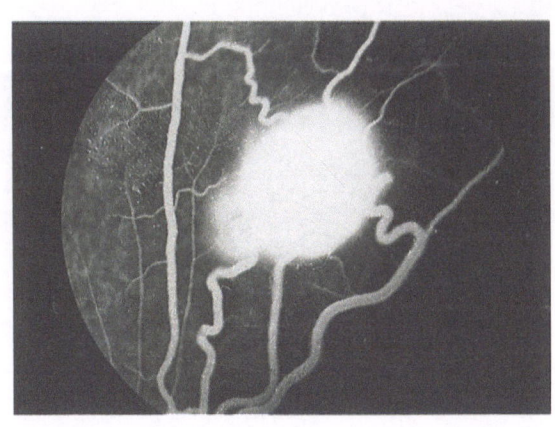

FIGURE 48-3.
Fluorescein angiogram depicts the shunting of arteriolar blood and venous blood in a hemangioma.

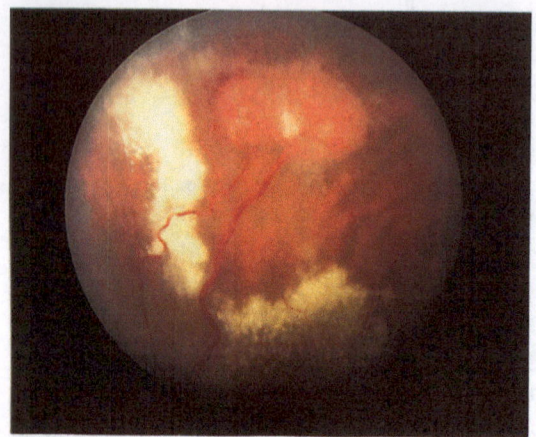

FIGURE 48-4.
As the tumors progress over time, they not only may enlarge but exhibit both intraretinal and subretinal exudation. (Courtesy of Dennis B. Freilich, M.D.)

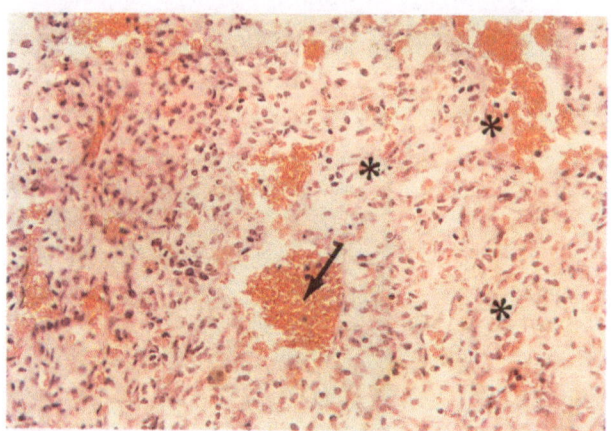

FIGURE 48-5.
Histopathology of a capillary hemangioma shows capillary vessels (arrow) filled with blood. Note the large number of endothelial cells. (H & E) (asterisks)

Chapter 49

Wyburn-Mason Syndrome (Racemose Hemangioma)

In Wyburn-Mason disorder there are arteriovenous communications of the retina and brain that begin during adolescence or early adulthood. Patients may demonstrate a visual loss, strabismus, pulsating exophthalmos, and ptosis. The racemose aneurysm of the retina is accompanied by an arteriovenous malformation in the brain. The communication is between an artery and a vein, bypassing a capillary bed. Intracranial calcifications can be seen on radiographic studies, and perivascular retinal atrophy can be demonstrated on fluorescein angiography. Systemic clinical manifestations include epilepsy, neurological defects, and intracranial hemorrhage. The retinal aneurysms are ipsilateral to the cranial lesions and do not have an associated exudation in the retina.

Selected Reading

Archer DB, Deutman A, Ernest JT, Krill AE (1973). Arteriovenous communications of the retina. Am J Ophthalmol 75:224-241

Wyburn-Mason R (1943). Arteriovenous aneurysm of midbrain and retina: facial nevi and mental changes. Brain 66:163-203

Figures

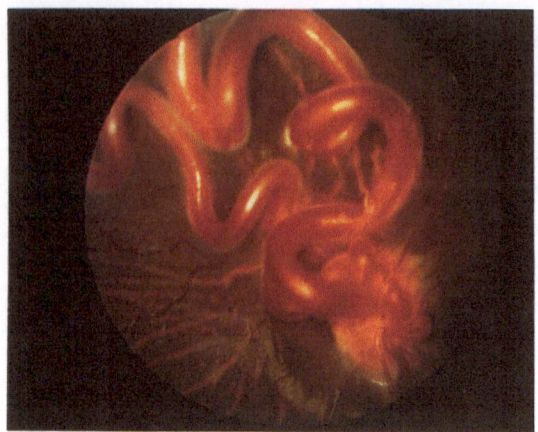

FIGURE 49-1.
Racemose angioma. The large vessels exit and enter at the disc.

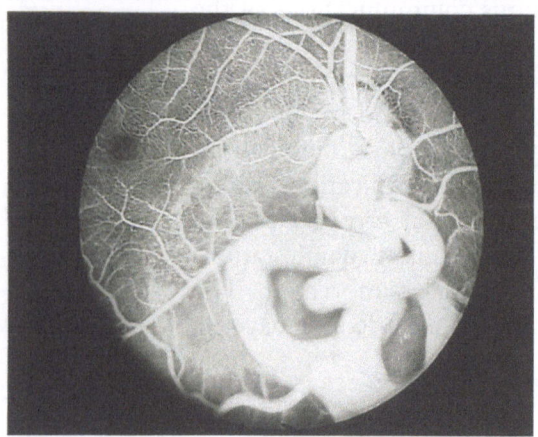

FIGURE 49-2.
Fluorescein angiography fills all the vessels evenly. The macula appears to be uninvolved. Note the loss of the normal capillary bed adjacent to the "aneurysmally" dilated vessel.

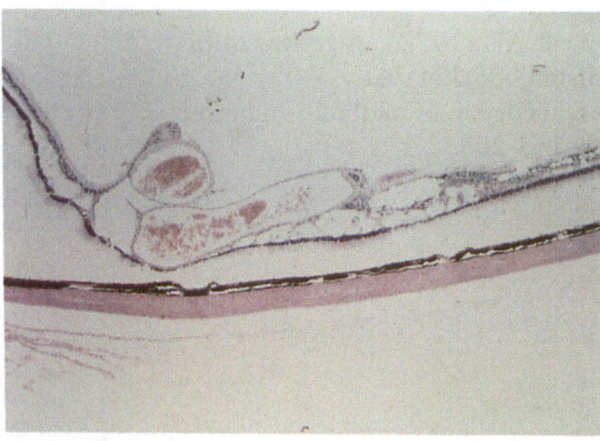

FIGURE 49-3.
Histopathology demonstrates dilated thin-walled vessels with atrophy of the adjacent retina. (H & E)

Section 10

Tumors

Chapter 50

Choroidal Nevi

A choroidal nevus usually is small, gray to brown, and oval or circular with feathery margins at times but usually with sharp borders. Nevi are usually flat, although they may have attained some height over time. Their size can vary from 0.5 mm to more than 5.0 mm in diameter. On fluorescein angiography, they block fluorescence. Visual field examination can demonstrate a scotoma. They usually have altered pigment on their surface.

Choroidal nevi exist in up to 6% of the general population. It is estimated that 1 of 5000 people with a nevus eventually will have a melanoma. Histology demonstrates that most nevi are composed of spindle cells.

Selected Reading

Ganley JP, Comstock GW (1973). Benign nevi and malignant melanomas of the choroid. Am J Ophthalmol 76:19-25

Figures

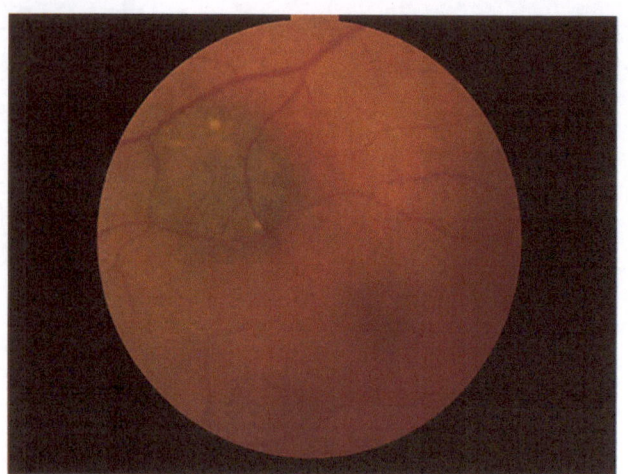

FIGURE 50-1.
This pigmented lesion is located under the vessels and has multiple drusen overlying it. It is avascular and flat. Most nevi are located in the posterior portion of the globe.

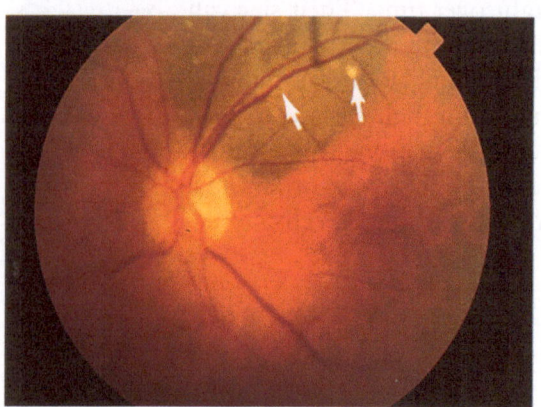

FIGURE 50-2.
Nevi may become large. Although nevi are typically approximately 0.5 disc diameter in size, this nevus has grown to almost 3.0 disc diameters. Note the drusen on its surface. (arrows)

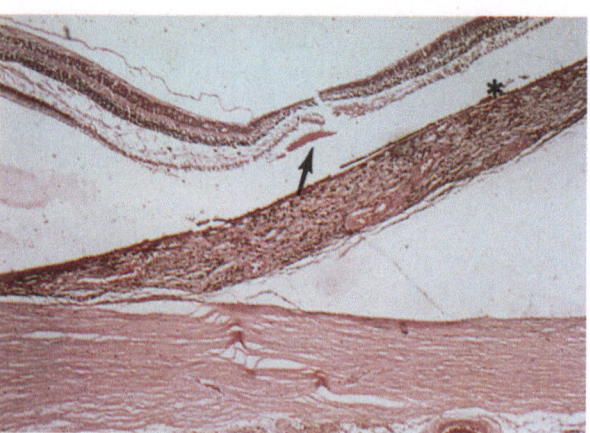

FIGURE 50-3.
Nevus of the choroid adjacent to the macula. Note the overlying serous detachment (arrow) of the sensory retina and the drusen underneath Bruch's membrane. (asterisk) (H & E)

Chapter 51

Melanocytoma of the Optic Nerve Head

A melanocyte may give rise to a melanocytoma, a benign, usually black tumor most commonly seen on or adjacent to the optic nerve. Histopathologically, the melanocytoma is a magnocellular nevus. Melanocytomas are probably present at birth, although the diagnosis is usually made later in life. They usually appear unilaterally, and there is no preferential predilection for women over men. Darkly pigmented individuals are more likely to be affected.

These masses are mostly jet-black with a feathered edge because the pigmented polyhedral cells travel into the nerve fiber layer. The tumors may be small or large, and they may sit on the edge of the disc or totally obscure it. An afferent pupillary defect is sometimes seen in large tumors. Rarely, large melanocytomas undergo necrosis or produce a vascular occlusion and lead to visual loss. In rare cases these masses undergo malignant transformation. Large melanocytomas may also alter surrounding retinal pigment epithelium and demonstrate sheathing of the disc vessels.

Fluorescein angiography demonstrates a hypofluorescent structure without intrinsic vasculature. The lesion is adjacent to or on the disc, so the visual field demonstrates an enlarged blind spot that may increase in size as the tumor enlarges. No therapy is necessary.

Histologically, melanocytomas are large, globular, polyhedral cells filled with pigment.

Selected Reading

Osher RH, Shields JA, Layman PR (1979). Pupillary and visual field evaluation in patients with melanocytoma of the optic disc. Arch Ophthalmol 97:1096-1099

Reidy JJ, Apple DJ, Steinmetz RL, et al (1985). Melanocytoma: nomenclature, pathogenesis, natural history and treatment. Surv Ophthalmol 29:319-327

Zimmerman LE (1965). Melanocytes, melanocytic nevi and melanocytomas. Invest Ophthalmol Vis Sci 4:11-41

Figures

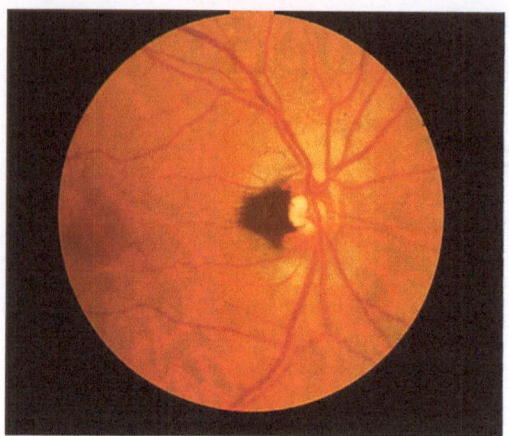

FIGURE 51-1.
Melanocytomas are composed of large polyhedral pigmented cells. They are characteristically black.

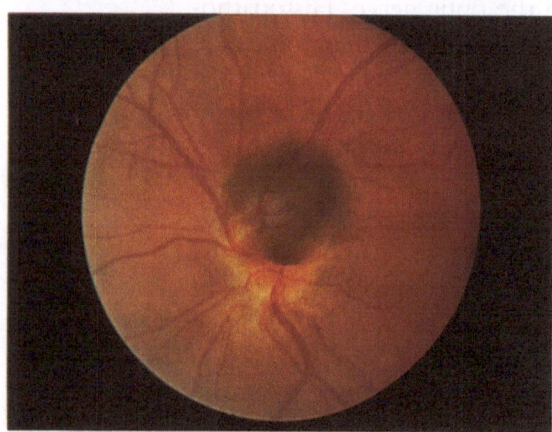

FIGURE 51-2.
Melanocytomas may become large, obscuring details of the disc. The lesion is most commonly seen in darkly pigmented patients.

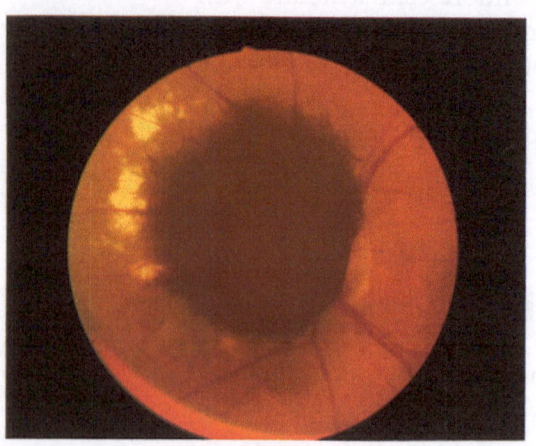

FIGURE 51-3.
Melanocytoma has grown and extends into overlying retina. Note the intraretinal exudation, a sign of growth.

FIGURE 51-4.
Histopathology of a melanocytoma reveals a large pigmented tumor involving the anterior portion of the optic nerve. (H & E)

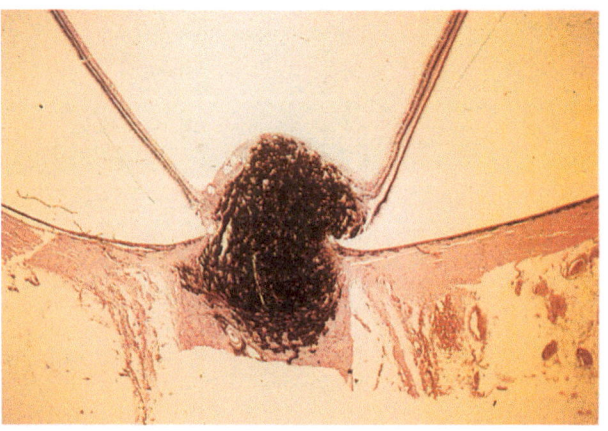

FIGURE 51-4.

Chapter 52

Melanoma

Uveal melanomas are not usually seen in the young adult; they are considered adult cancers. The lesion is likewise unusual in blacks, native Americans and Americans of Oriental extraction. Blue irides, male gender, and exposure to prolonged sunlight are some of the factors commonly seen in patients with melanoma of the choroid.

Ophthalmoscopy alone correctly identifies a melanoma in 95% of cases. The melanoma can be mushroom-shaped, have orange pigment on its surface, have an exudative detachment overlying the tumor, and be elevated and globular in shape, arising from the choroid. Melanomas do not usually hemorrhage unless they have been treated with photocoagulation. Up to 25% of these tumors are amelanotic. Black pigmentation is not seen with melanomas. There is usually no inflammatory component with a melanoma.

Fluorescein angiography demonstrates hot spots within the tumor as well as an intratumoral circulation. Imaging can be done with B-scan ultrasonography, magnetic resonance imaging, or computed tomography. Quantitative echography also gives a more accurate diagnosis than the routine B-scan. The B-scan demonstrates an excavation of the choroid, a quiet zone, and orbital shadowing. Fine-needle aspiration biopsy can assist with the diagnosis of medium-sized melanomas.

Therapeutic suggestions have been plentiful. Xenon arc or argon laser photocoagulation, radioactive plaques, charged particle irradiation, surgical resection, and enucleation have all been utilized to treat these tumors. Systemic evaluation prior to any therapy is essential to rule out metastasis.

Histologically, melanomas arise de novo from melanocytes and preexisting nevus cells of the choroid. The spindle A-cell type accounts for 5% of all melanomas with 92% five-year survival. Mitotic figures are rarely seen. The nuclei are associated with a folding of the nuclear membrane, giving rise to a nuclear stripe. The spindle B-cell and fascicular types account for approximately 40% of all melanomas. Spindle B-cells have a prominent nucleus. The 5-year survival is 70%. The mixed-cell type (spindle B-cells and epithelioid) tumors account for 45% of melanomas and are associated with a 41% five-year survival rate. The epithelioid type accounts for 5% of the tumors.

Mitotic rates are common, and the 5-year survival is 30%. Necrotic tumors account for 7% of tumors and have a 5-year survival of 41%.

Selected Reading

Augsberger JJ, Games JW, Sardi VF, et al (1986). Enucleation vs cobalt plaque radiotherapy for malignant melanomas of the choroid and ciliary body. Arch Ophthalmol 104:655-661

Gragoudas ES, Seddon J, Goitein M, et al (1985). Current results of proton beam irradiation of uveal melanomas. Ophthalmology 92:284-291

Meyer-Schwickerath G, Vogel MH (1974). Treatment of malignant melanomas treated with photocoagulation: a ten year follow up. Mod Probl Ophthalmol 12:544-549

Orellana J, McPherson AR (1984). Treatment of medium sized malignant melanomas. Ann Ophthalmol 16:412-416

Peyman GH, Juarez CP, Diamond JG, Raichand M (1984). Ten years' experience with eye wall resection for uveal malignant melanomas. Ophthalmology 91:1720-1725

Shields CL, Shields JA, Milite J, et al (1991). Uveal melanoma in teenagers and children: a report of 40 cases. Ophthalmology 98:1662-1666

Shields JA, Rodrigues MM, Sarin LK, et al (1976). Lipofuscin pigment over benign and malignant choroidal tumors. Trans Am Acad Ophthalmol Otolaryngol 81:871-881

Figures

FIGURE 52-1.
Medium-sized malignant melanoma located in the posterior pole. It has grown over 3 years after exhibiting no growth for the previous 10 years.

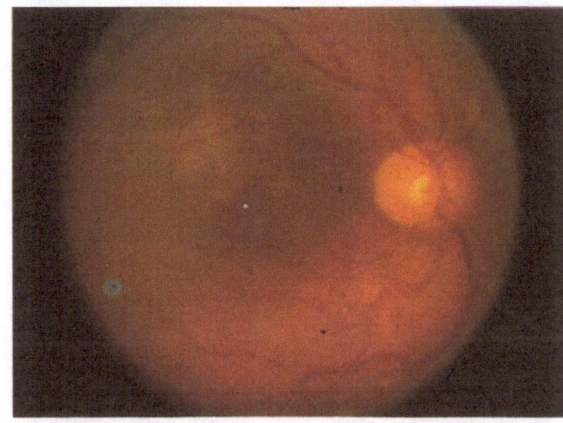

FIGURE 52-2.
This patient noted the growth of "something on my iris" over 2 years. The angle was occluded by the tumor from 7 to 11 o'clock. Iris melanomas account for fewer than 10% of all uveal melanomas, and they arise from preexisting nevi.

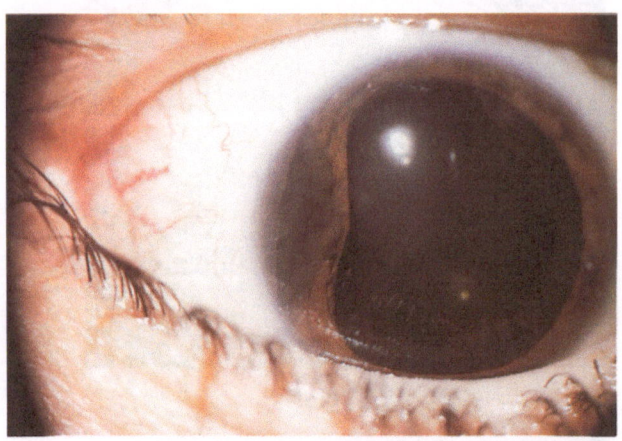

FIGURE 52-3.
Large melanoma (diameter >10 mm, height >5 mm). There is an overlying serous retinal detachment.

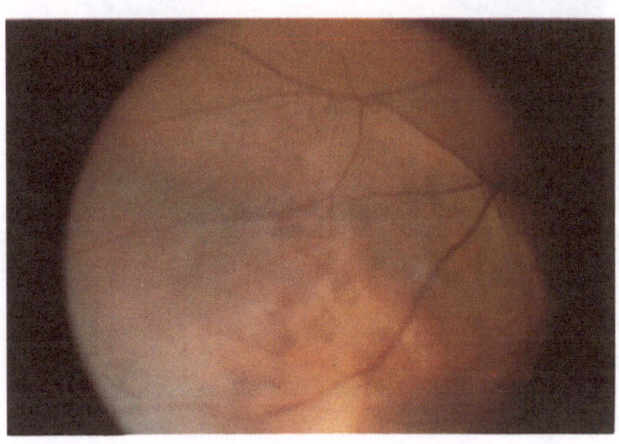

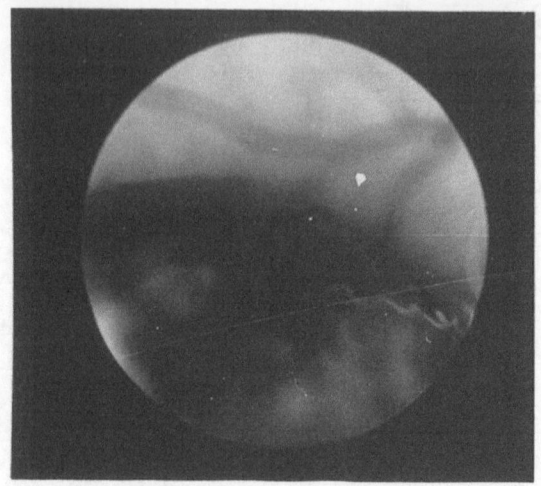

A

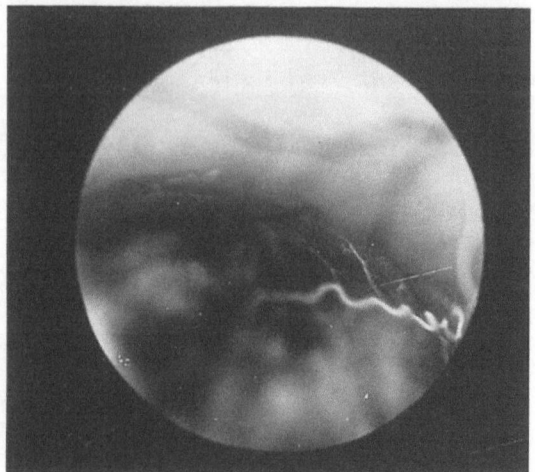

B

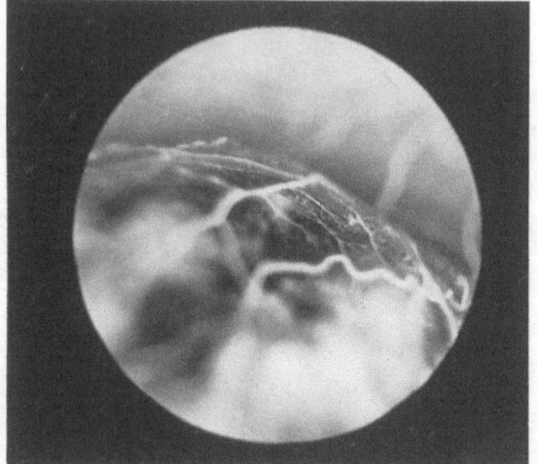

C

FIGURE 52-4.
(A) Retinal vessels appear over the tumor mass. (B) Mottled fluorescence is seen within the tumor. (C) Fluorescence returns to the mass—a double circulation is present.

FIGURE 52-5.
In this gross specimen, we can see that a choroidal mass has broken through Bruch's membrane. A serous detachment is also present.

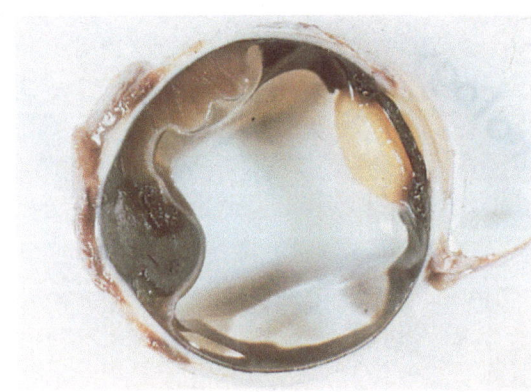

FIGURE 52-6.
Spindle A cells are extensive. There are no nucleoli in these cells. They contain a central dark stripe that corresponds to a nuclear fold. (H & E)

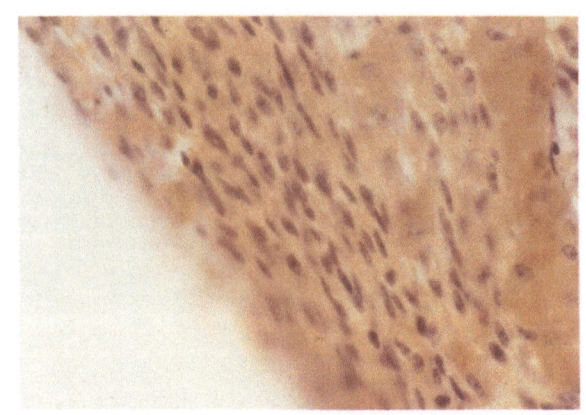

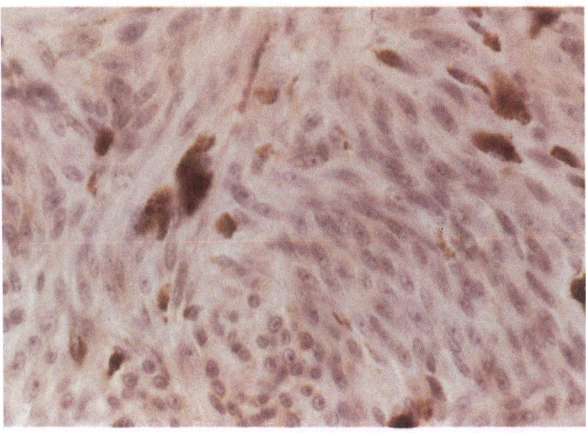

FIGURE 52-7.
Spindle B cells. They have indistinct cell borders and possess nucleoli. (H & E)

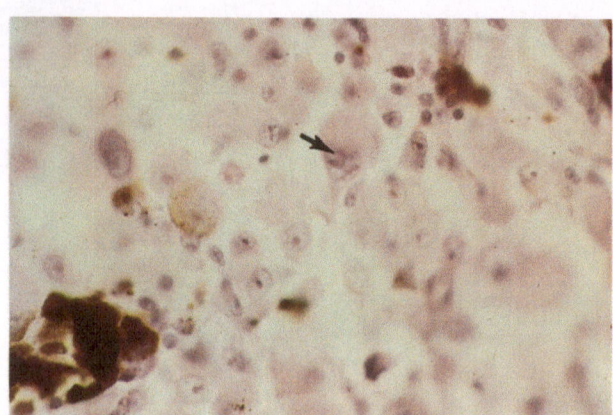

FIGURE 52-8.
Unlike spindle A- and B-cells, which are cohesive, these cells are not. They are epithelioid (arrow) and have distinct cell borders and prominent nucleoli. (H & E)

Chapter 53

Medulloepithelioma

A medulloepithelioma, or diktyoma, is a congenital tumor of the ciliary body. The prefix medullo- suggests that its origin is in the medullary epithelium, which not only lines the neural tube but also forms the primitive bilayered optic cup. Medulloepitheliomas can also arise from iris, optic nerve, or retina. They are congenital, unilateral tumors that display no evidence of genetic transmission. Affected children present with a loss of vision during the first decade of life with a mass in the ciliary body, glaucoma, or cataract. Medulloepitheliomas can be classified as teratoid or nonteratoid, with each type further divided into benign or malignant. They are, for the most part, slow-growing tumors that usually do not metastasize. In adults, medulloepitheliomas can be malignant.

Histologically, these tumors are composed of the cords of epithelium and a matrix. The epithelial cells may be separated into pigmented and nonpigmented cells. The matrix resembles embyonic matrix or primary vitreous, staining positively for the presence of hyaluronic acid.

Selected Reading

Hamburg A (1980). Medulloepithelioma arising from the posterior pole. Ophthalmologica 181:152-159

Orellana J, Moura RA, Font RL, et al (1983). Medulloepithelioma diagnosed by ultrasound and vitreous aspirate: electron microscopic observations. Ophthalmology 90:1531-1539

Figures

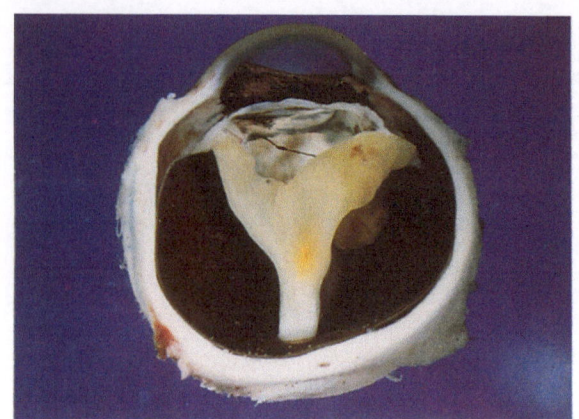

FIGURE 53-1.
This child had no light perception and a medulloepithelioma of the ciliary body. A chord of pigmented cells traverses the vitreous cavity. (Courtesy of Ophthalmology) Orellana J, Moura RA, Font RL

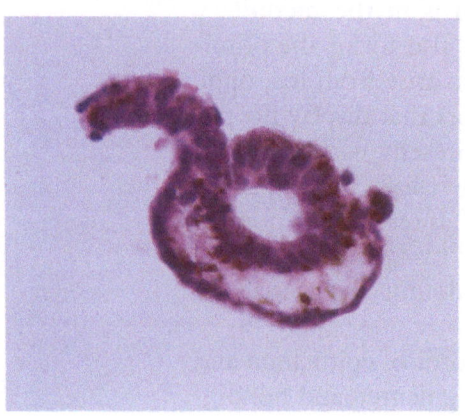

FIGURE 53-2.
Medulloepitheliomas can contain areas where undifferentiated cells reside. Other areas may contain cells resembling rosettes. Here we see such a rosette. (H & E) (Courtesy of Ophthalmology Orellana J, Moura RA, Font RL, et al Ophthalmology 1983 90:1531-1539)

Chapter 54

Retinoblastoma

Although most retinoblastomas are not inherited, they do demonstrate an autosomal dominant inheritance pattern. Unilateral cases tend to be sporadic in origin, whereas bilateral cases are genetically determined. Retinoblastoma is the most common malignant tumor of childhood and many investigators believe that its incidence is increasing.

The most common presenting sign is leukocoria, followed by strabismus, evidence of intraocular inflammation, visual loss, mydriasis, pseudohypopyon, and occasionally vitreous hemorrhage. Development of a cataract is unusual. Endophytic tumors grow toward the vitreous, and tumors that grow toward the choroid are termed exophytic. The Reese-Ellsworth classification is used to classify these tumors into groups. Patients with unilateral disease should be followed closely, as the incidence of fellow eye tumors approaches 20%. Trilateral retinoblastoma refers to bilateral disease along with a pinealoblastoma. Morphology of the pinealoblastoma resembles that of the retinoblastoma. It is located in the pineal gland, which in lower vertebrates has photoreceptor as well as endocrine functions. (It is present in humans as well.)

Retinoblastomas can also be the result of chromosomal deletion. An example is deletion of band 14 on chromosome 13, that is, a deletion on the long arm of chromosome 13. Such children have retinoblastomas accompanied by mental retardation and facial anomalies. The ratio of unilateral/bilateral retinoblastomas in this syndrome is the same as in regular retinoblastoma populations. All bilateral retinoblastoma patients are at risk of developing secondary malignancies, such as osteogenic sarcoma of the orbit or femur. This tendency may be carried by the retinoblastoma gene, and the possiblity of a secondary malignancy increases if the patient was exposed to radiation.

Ultrasonography can demonstrate calcifications within the eye, corresponding to calcification of the tumorous mass. Because tumors leak fluorescein, this substance can be helpful for determining whether a retinal mass is an astrocytic hamartoma or a retinoblastoma. Endophytic tumor destruction yields a mass that no longer leaks fluorescein. Cytological

229

examination of the aqueous may be useful, as may assay of lactic dehydrogenase levels in both plasma and aqueous. Computed tomography (CT) or magnetic resonance imaging is needed in children with bilateral retinoblastomas.

Selected Reading

Jensen RD, Miller RW (1971). Retinoblastoma: epidemiological characteristics. N Engl J Med 285:307-311

Messmer EP, Heinrich T, Hopping W, et al (1991). Risk factors for metastasis in patients with retinoblastoma. Ophthalmology 98:136-141

Shields CL, Shields JA, Shah P (1991). Retinoblastoma in older children. Ophthalmology 98:395-399

Shields JA, Sanborn GE, Augsberger JJ, et al (1982). Fluorescein angiography of retinoblastoma. Trans Am Ophthalmol Soc 80:98-112

Vogel F (1979). Genetics of retinoblastoma. Hum Genet 52:1-54

Figures

FIGURE 54-1.
This young boy has the white reflex seen with retinoblastoma. The child's mother noted the reflex on several photographs and took the child to a pediatrician.

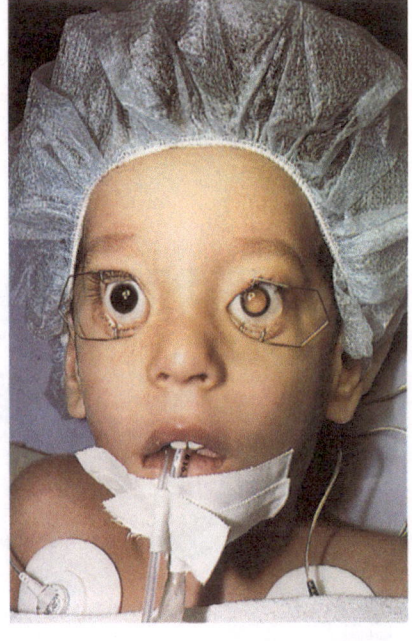

FIGURE 54-2.
On enucleation, the tumor occupies 50% of the posterior cavity, abutting the inferior portion of the lens.

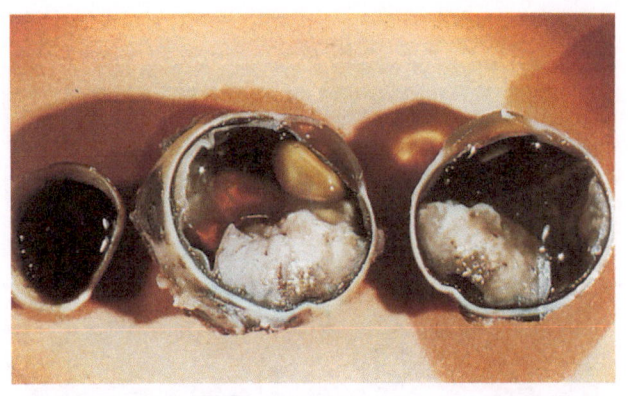

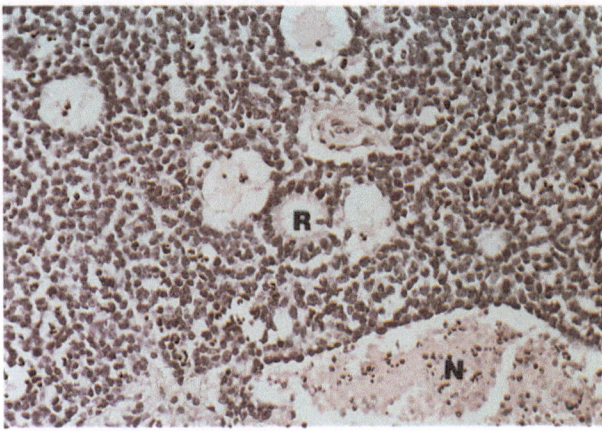

FIGURE 54-3.
Rosettes. (H & E) (R) Note area of necrosis (N).

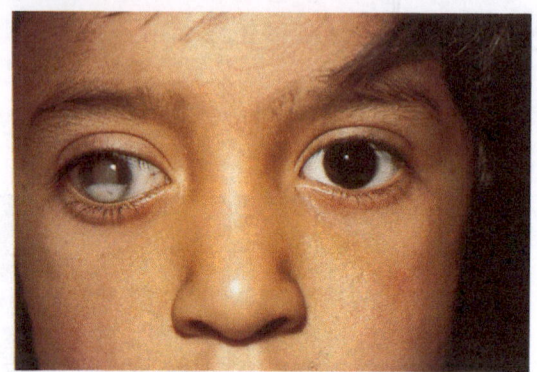

FIGURE 54-4.
This child was referred from Peru for a pseudohypopyon that had been present for 3 months. The child underwent enucleation and radiotherapy. She also received a full course of chemotherapy in Lima, Peru. Eight years later, she is alive and doing well.

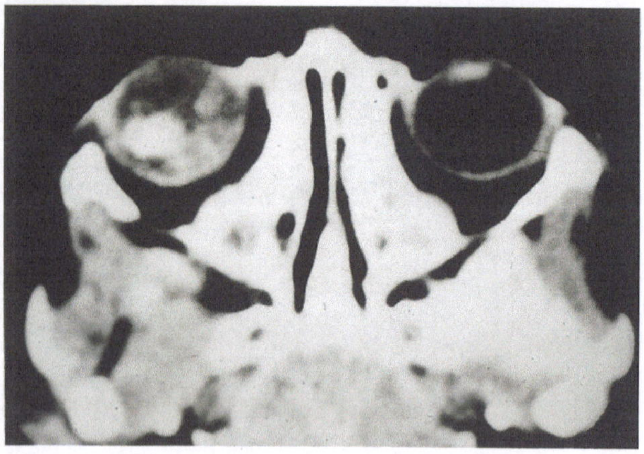

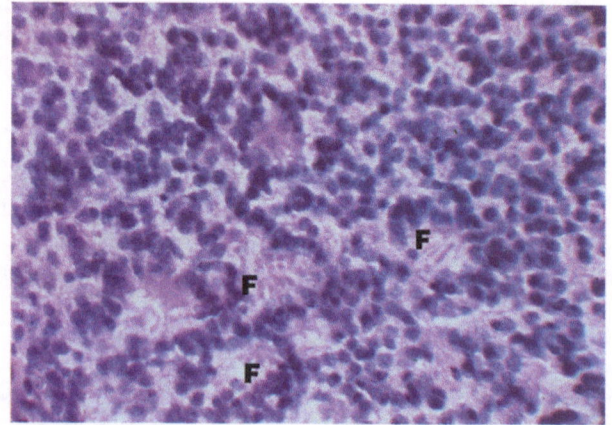

FIGURE 54-5.
CT scan of the patient in Fig. 54-4 demonstrates a tumor-filled eye.

FIGURE 54-6.
Histopathology demonstrates multiple fleurettes (F) in the field, indicating photoreceptor differentiation within the tumor. (H & E)

FIGURE 54-7.
This specimen was from a 2-year-old child. The tumor shows undifferentiated cells. (H & E)

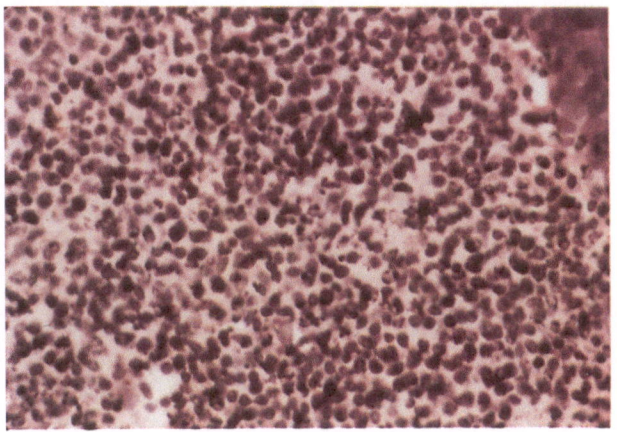

Section 11

Miscellaneous Disorders

Section 14

Miscellaneous Disorders

Chapter 55

Albinism

The paucity of melanin in the usually pigmented tissues of hair, skin, and eyes comprises the syndrome of oculocutaneous albinism. The patient population can be subdivided into those with a permanent lack of melanin (tyrosinase-negative) and those who have some melanin (tyrosinase-positive). If the eyes alone are affected, the syndrome is called ocular albinism. There are at least ten types of oculocutaneous albinism and four types of ocular albinism.

In patients with oculocutaneous albinism, the clinical picture is striking. Characteristically, the child has white skin and a pink iris that easily transilluminates. The absence of fundus pigmentation produces a blond fundus without xanthophyllic pigmentation at the fovea. The optic nerve can be hypoplastic, and the patients usually exhibit nystagmus with decreased visual acuity.

The fluorescein angiogram can confirm the paucity of melanin. The study demonstrates multiple transmission defects in retinal pigment epithelium with little melanin or a sheet of translucency due to no melanin. A specific type of oculocutaneous albinism is the Hermansky-Pudlak syndrome. These patients have varying amounts of pigmentation with the typical signs of albinism. They also have a hemorrhagic diathesis and abnormal reticular cells in the bone marrow. Such patients must be cautious about ingesting aspirin or indomethacin, as it interferes with an already abnormal hematological condition. The condition is autosomal recessive in inheritance. The electroretinogram (ERG) may be normal or show a modest decrease in rod and cone responses. With other types of oculocutaneous albinism, the ERG is larger and faster than normal. The visually evoked responses demonstrate a rewiring effect in that a P 100 wave can often be elicited in the contralateral scalp.

Ocular albinism is a separate entity in which the skin and hair are apparently normal. The patients have nystagmus and decreased pigmentation of the ocular tissues. Genetically, the disorder is X-linked. The patients have photophobia, nystagmus, and poor acuity. The iris may be blue or hazel, or it may even darken during young adulthood. Female carriers have patchy areas of pigmentation confirmed by fluorescein angiography. Skin biopsy identifies the patient as having ocular albinism. Treatment is similar for all these patients. They may require strabismus surgery, tinted lenses, and careful refraction to attain the best possible acuity.

Selected Reading

Hermansky F, Pudlak P (1959). Albinism associated with hemorrhagic diathesis and unusual pigmented reticular cells in the bone marrow: report of two cases with histochemical studies. Blood 14:162-169

Krill AE, Lee GB (1963). The electroretinogram in albinos and carriers of the ocular albino trait. Arch Ophthalmol 69:32-38

Simon JW, Adams RJ, Calhoun JH, et al (1982). Ophthalmic manifestations of the Hermansky-Pudlak syndrome (oculocutaneous albinism and hemorrhagic diathesis). Am J Ophthalmol 93:71-77

Taylor WOG (1978). Visual disabilities of oculocutaneous albinism and their alleviation. Trans Ophthalmol Soc UK 98:423-445

Figures

FIGURE 55-1.
This boy has ocular albinism, inherited in an X-linked recessive manner. Note that the child has some pigmentation (he is black). His acuity is 20/200 in each eye, with nystagmus and photophobia.

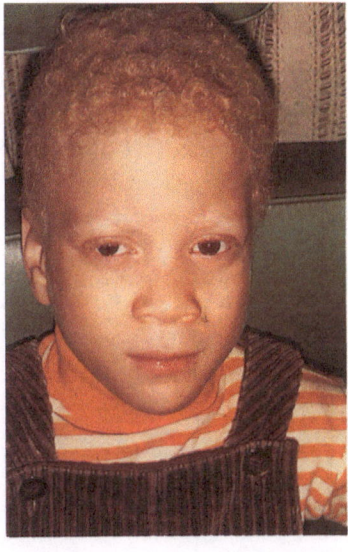

FIGURE 55-2.
Iris transillumination can easily be seen using the slit lamp.

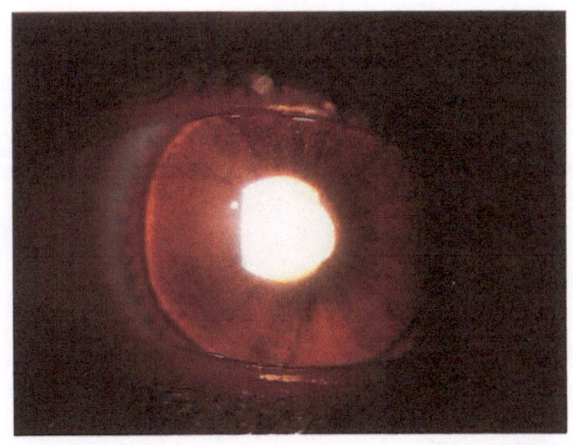

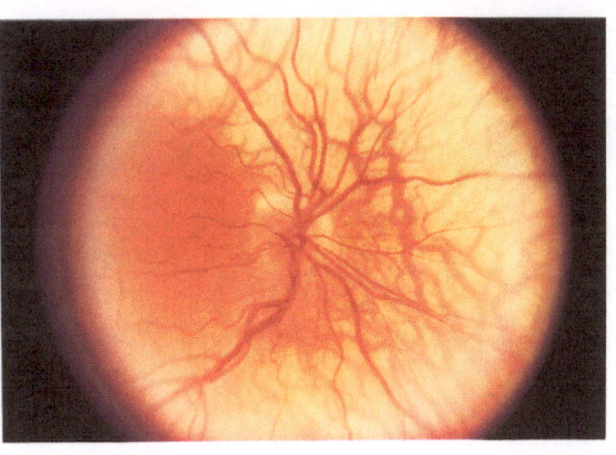

FIGURE 55-3.
Funduscopic evaluation produces a blond fundus with minimal pigmentation. The child had foveal aplasia, which causes the poor visual acuity.

Chapter 56

Angioid Streaks

Linear disruptions in Bruch's membranes that radiate outward from the optic nerve are called angioid streaks. Usually the breaks in Bruch's are seen as dull gray or green lesions that can radiate toward the periphery or straight to the fovea. There are several diseases or clinical entities that coexist with angioid streaks. The hereditary pattern of angioid streaks follows the hereditary pattern of the individual disease process. Typically, patients with pseudoxanthoma elasticum, Ehlers-Danlos syndrome, or Paget's disease exhibit angioid streaks.

The color vision is normal unless the associated disease has other ophthalmic problems associated with it. For example, sickle cell patients who have been extensively treated with photocoagulation have an abnormality in their color vision. Electroretinography and electrooculography are normal. Fluorescein angiography delineates the lesions. The main complication of the streaks is subretinal neovascularization, which can be shown by fluorescein angiography.

Histopathologically, the gray-brown tissue interrupts the basophilia of Bruch's membrane. Fibrovascular tissue may be present at these breaks, especially when clinical neovascularization is present. The retinal pigment epithelium may be abnormal.

Selected Reading

Gass JDM, Clarkson JG (1973). Angioid streaks and disciform macular detachment in Paget's disease (osteitis deformans). Am J Ophthalmol 75:576-586

Green WR, Friedman-Kien A, Banfield WG (1966). Angioid streaks in Ehlers-Danlos syndrome. Arch Ophthalmol 76:197-204

Smith JL, Gass JDM, Justice J (1964). Fluorescein fundus photography of angioid streaks. Br J Ophthalmol 48:517-521

Figures

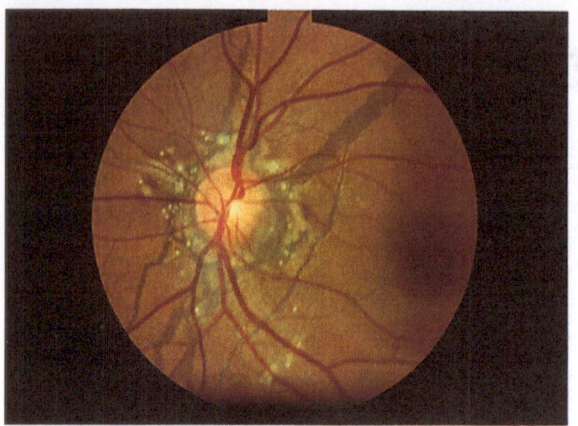

FIGURE 56-1.
Typical irregular radiating angioid streaks. The streaks are caused by breaks in the collagenous layer of Bruch's membrane.

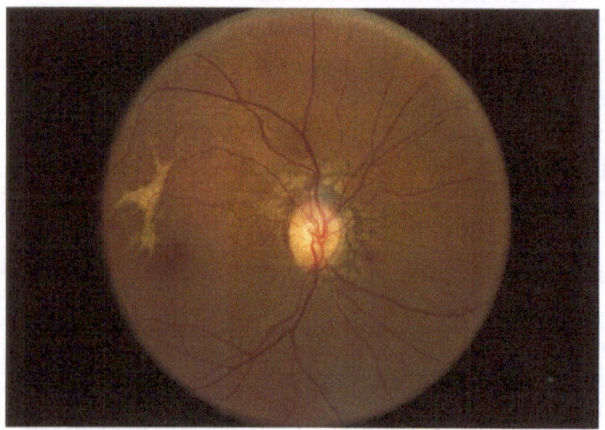

FIGURE 56-2.
Angioid streaks situated around the optic nerve. In addition, there is a crack through the macula. Often a choroidal neovascular membrane begins under these cracks in Bruch's membrane. Hemorrhagic detachment of the RPE may ensue. Trauma can also be the cause of sudden visual loss when a choroidal rupture or submacular hemorrhage occurs.

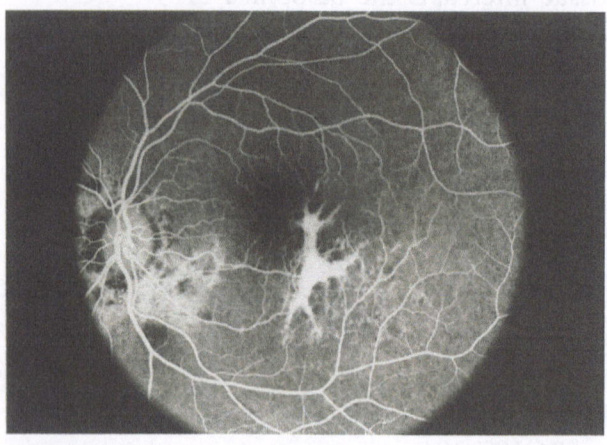

FIGURE 56-3.
Fluorescein angiogram demonstrating the peripapillary changes seen in patients with angioid streaks. More impressive is the break in Bruch's seen at the macula. Such lesions are often associated with the development of subretinal membranes.

FIGURE 56-4.
Pseudoxanthoma elasticum. Note the basophilia of Bruch's membrane with a prominent break (toward the right) and proliferation of fibrous tissue (arrow) from the choroid through the break. (H & E)

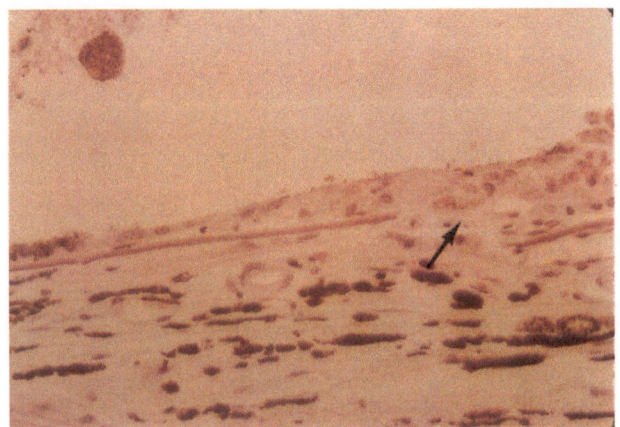

Chapter 57

Incontinentia Pigmenti (Bloch-Sulzberger Syndrome)

Incontinentia pigmenti is not common. It is X-linked dominant and is lethal in most affected male infants. Usually the males with the disease are stillborn. There are dermal, central nervous system, ocular, and dental involvements with this disease.

The skin lesions progress through several stages. At birth the skin has blisters that give rise to warty outgrowths. These growths then subside and become hyperpigmented whorls, which may remain for life. Ocular problems are seen in about one-third of patients. Some of the more serious causes of vision loss in these patients include cataracts, retinal neovascularization, chorioretinitis, uveitis, pseudoglioma, retinal detachment, optic atrophy, and a combination of these problems. Strabismus and nystagmus can also occur. Some investigators have reported whorls of pigment in the fundus.

The skin histopathology shows macrophages containing dystrophic cells and melanosome complexes. In the blister stage, eosinophilia may be associated.

Selected Readings

Carney RG (1976). Incontinentia pigmenti: a world statistical analysis. Arch Dermatol 112:535-542

Wilund DA, Weston WL (1980). Incontinentia pigmenti. Arch Dermatol 116:701-703

Figures

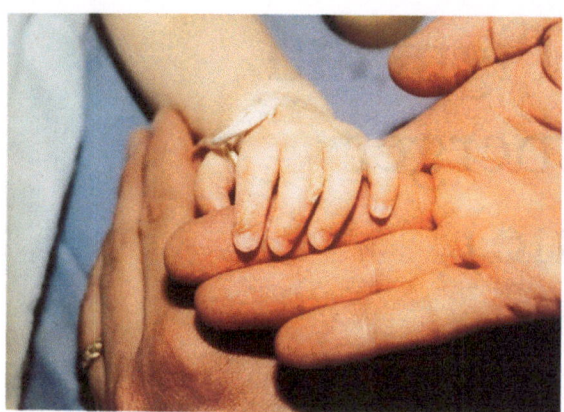

FIGURE 57-1.
Warty outgrowths follow resolution of the blisters at 6 weeks. Here the warts can be seen on the patient's fingers.

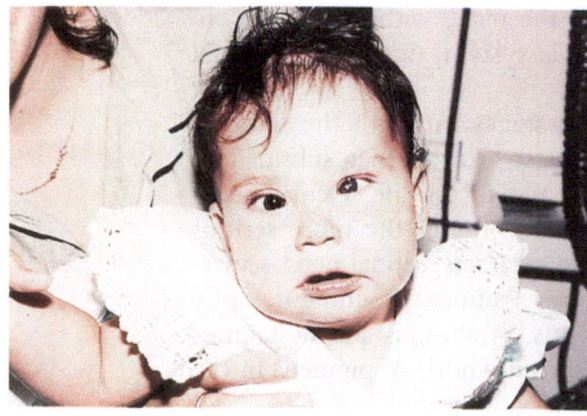

FIGURE 57-2.
Strabismus and a pseudoglioma.

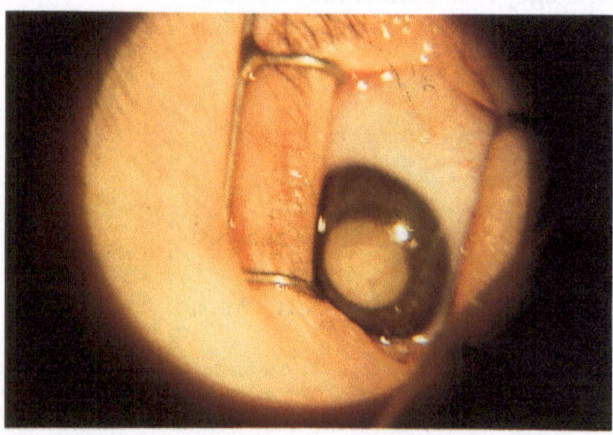

FIGURE 57-3.
Left eye has an opacity behind the lens that is vascular. Ultrasonography showed total detachment.

FIGURE 57-4.
Note hyperpigmented whorls on the leg seen in these children. These whorls can either resolve or remain for the life of the patient.

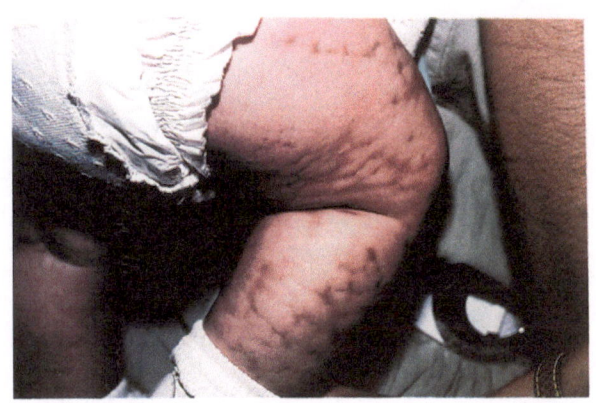

Chapter 58

Myelinated Nerve Fibers

Myelination proceeds in an orderly fashion. The last elements to receive a myelin sheath are the chiasm and optic nerve. Myelinated nerve fibers in the retina most often occur in men and are seen in 0.3-1.0% of individuals. The eyes are otherwise normal.

On histology, the patches located within the nerve fiber layer stain for myelin. Despite the dramatic appearance, the eye is otherwise normal in most cases. A scotoma can be seen on visual field testing in some patients. Demyelination has been reported with multiple sclerosis.

Selected Reading

Magoon EH, Robb RM (1981). Development of myelin in human optic nerve and tract: a light and electron microscopic study. Arch Ophthalmol 99:655-659

Straatsma BR, Foos RY, Heekenlively JR et al (1981). Myelinated retinal nerve fibers. Am J Ophthalmol 91:25-38

Figures

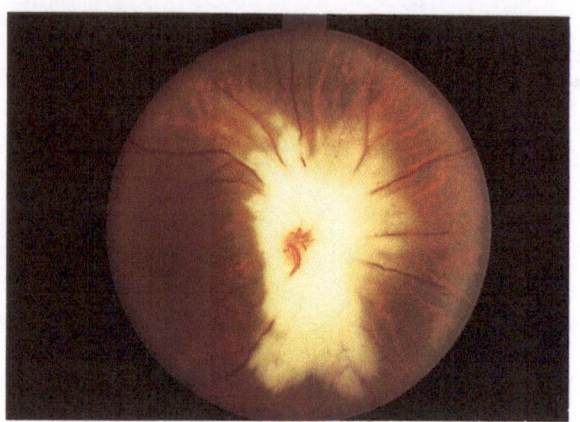

FIGURE 58-1.
These lesions are striking and nonprogressive. The yellow-white patches run in the nerve fiber layer and appear to be emanating from the disc.

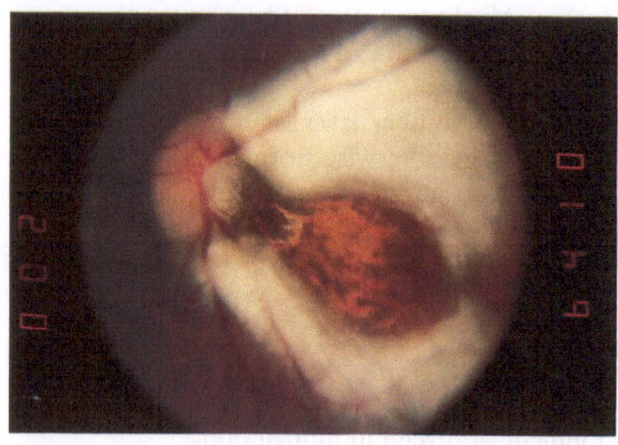

FIGURE 58-2.
Retinal myelinated nerve fibers. Patients with such extensive myelination often have ipsilateral myopia. This patient's refraction was -8.50. (Courtesy of Ronni M. Lieberman, M.D.)

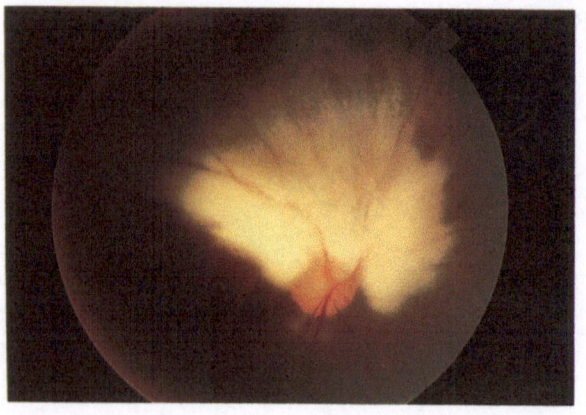

FIGURE 58-3.
It is not unusual to see extensive myelination, as in this case, superior to the optic disc.

FIGURE 58-4.
Myelinated nerve fibers need not originate at the disc margins. In this patient, myelination occurred at a distance from the optic disc.

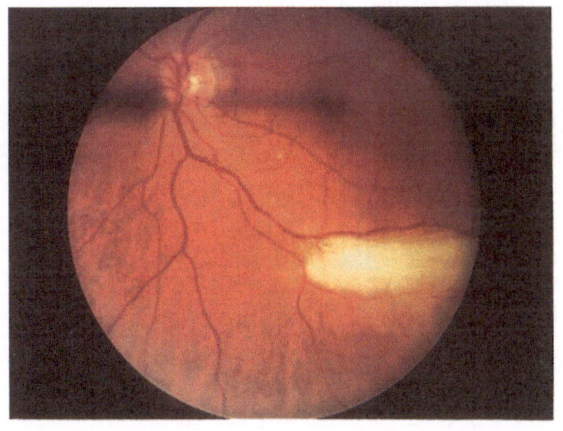

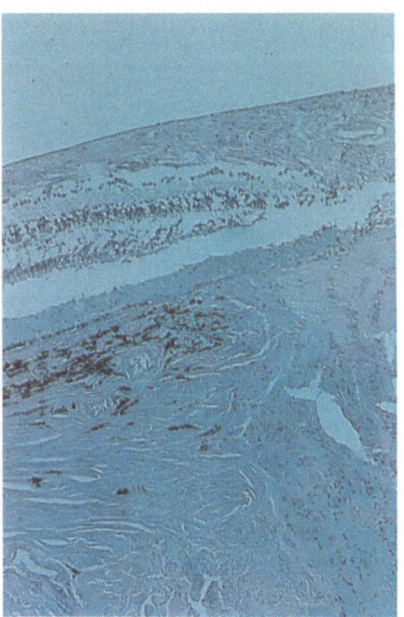

FIGURE 58-5.
Myelin. (Luxol fast blue)

Chapter 59

Myopia

Simple myopia is a commonly encountered variation in refraction. It is determined via a polygenic mode of inheritance. Myopia can be simple; much more devastating, however, is degenerative myopia where several pathological changes occur in the eye. The length of the eye enlarges and is associated with progressive thinning of the sclera. Ultimately, the sclera thins and a staphyloma appears at the posterior pole. Staphylomas readily occur in eyes with an axial length of more than 26.5 mm. Staphylomas are invariably associated with decreased visual acuity. A thinning choroid and disappearing choriocapillaris are seen in eyes with degenerative myopia. The visual field can demonstrate an enlarged blind spot or scotomas. The ERG can be normal or subnormal while the EOG is normal. Lacquer cracks and temporal disc crescents are other signs of degenerative myopia. Because of breaks in Bruch's membrane, subretinal neovascular nets frequently develop at the fovea. The hyperpigmentation seen at the fovea after a bleed is called a Fuch's spot.

Open-angle glaucoma, vitreous liquefaction, lattice degeneration, retinal detachment, and cataracts seem to have a higher incidence in patients with myopia. Systemic disorders associated with myopia include retinopathy of prematurity, Marfan syndrome, Down syndrome, and Ehlers-Danlos syndrome. Histopathology demonstrates pigment epithelial and choriocapillaris atrophy. Photoreceptor degeneration can also be present.

Selected Reading

Curtin BJ (1970). Myopia: a review of its etiology, pathogenesis, and treatment. Surv Ophthalmol 15:1-17

Fuchs E (1901). Der zentrale schwarze Fleck bei Myopie. Z Augenheilkd 5:171-178

Figures

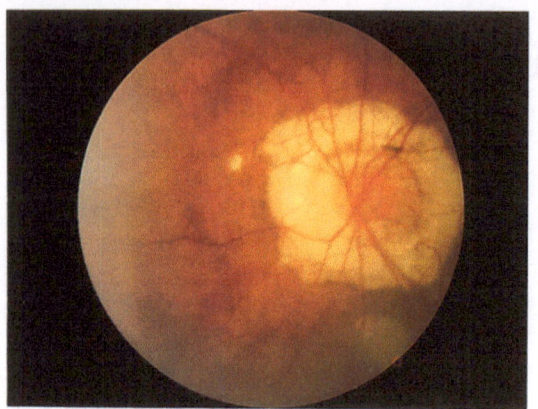

FIGURE 59-1
This patient has a refractive error of -14.50 diopters. Note the large peripapillary crescent that almost gives the appearance of having a small optic nerve head.

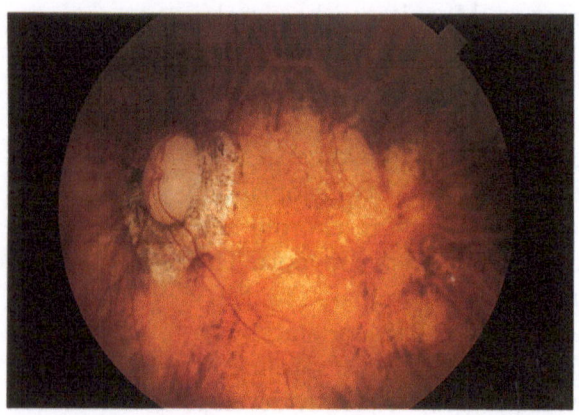

FIGURE 59-2.
Peripapillary crescent is present for 360 degrees in this patient. The retina is so atrophic and the RPE so attenuated that the choroidal vasculature is readily identified.

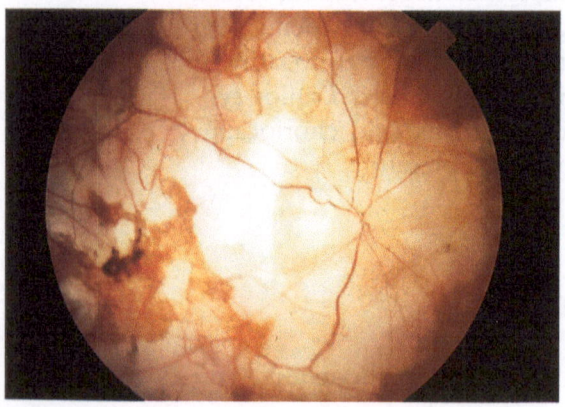

FIGURE 59-3.
Extensive myopic degeneration. Most of the fundus demonstrates foci of atrophy of the RPE and choroid due to the lacquer cracks.

FIGURE 59-4.
Fluorescein angiogram demonstrating the extensive loss of the RPE. The vasculature is attenuated owing to the excessive anteroposterior elongation of the globe.

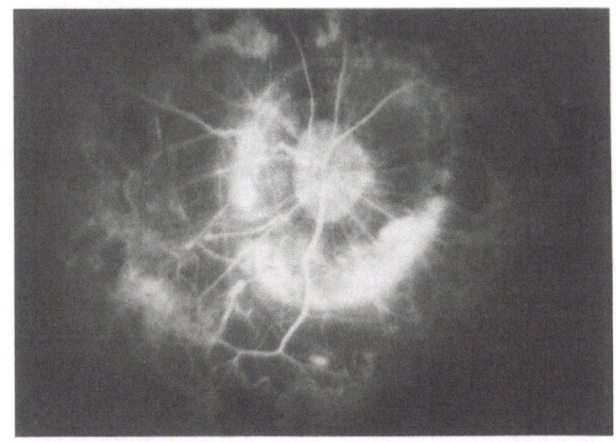

FIGURE 59-5.
This man suffered a subfoveal hemorrhage with a decrease of vision to count fingers. Two months later, the lesion at the fovea appeared as a small black dot. The visual acuity returned to 20/25.

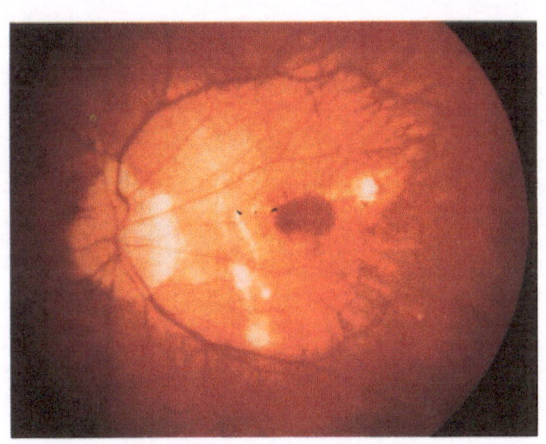

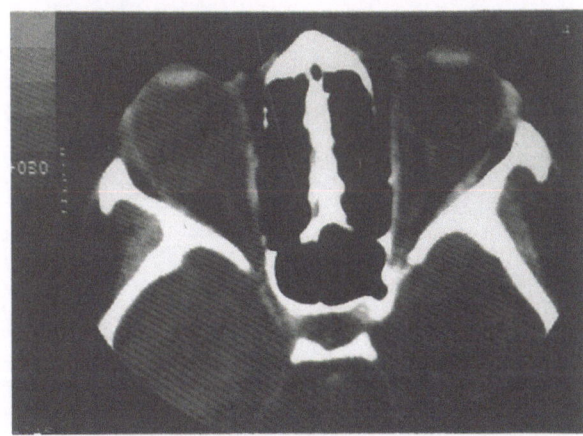

FIGURE 59-6.
This patient was noted to have "proptosis" by her internist. The patient insisted that her acuity in the right eye was always poor. CT scan shows that her "poorer" eye was considerably longer than the other eye. Axial myopia accounted for her "proptosis."

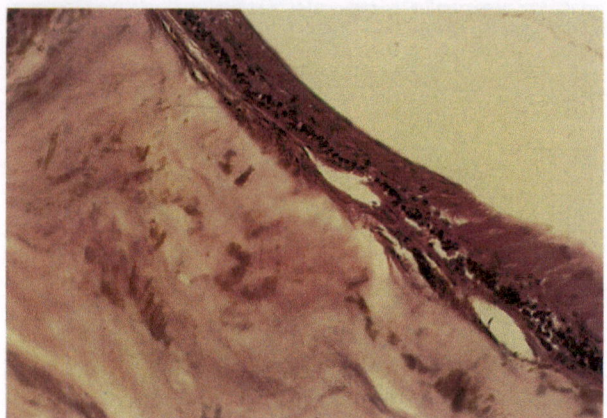

FIGURE 59-7.
Extensive atrophy of the choroid and retina due to extreme myopia. (H & E)

Chapter 60

Fabry's Disease

Fabry's disease, also called angiokeratoma corporis diffusum universale, is an X-linked recessive condition of males. It is due to an inborn error of glycolipid metabolism due to a deficiency of the enzyme α–galactosidase and where ceramide trihexose is stored in tissues. Typically, these patients have cutaneous angiokeratomas and whorl-like corneal dystrophy. Painful febrile episodes, renal failure, and cardiovascular disease develop. The accumulation of the ceramide trihexose in tissues creates the clinical picture. In addition to the corneal whorls, there are associated anterior and posterior capsular lens changes, conjunctival vascular changes, and a tortuosity of the retinal vasculature.

Histopathologically, there is deposition of the ceramide trihexose in all tissues. Endothelium, pericytes of retinal capillaries and choriocapillaries, and smooth muscle cells are preferentially involved. Electron microscopy of the retinal vasculature demonstrates lipoid deposits as well as osmophilic inclusion bodies.

Selected Reading

Font RL, Fine BS (1972). Ocular pathology in Fabry's disease—histochemical and electron microscopic observations. Am J Ophthalmol 73:419-430

Riegel EM, Pokorny KS, Friedman AH, et al (1982). Ocular pathology of Fabry's disease in a hemizygous male following renal transplantation. Surv Ophthalmol 26:247-252

Figures

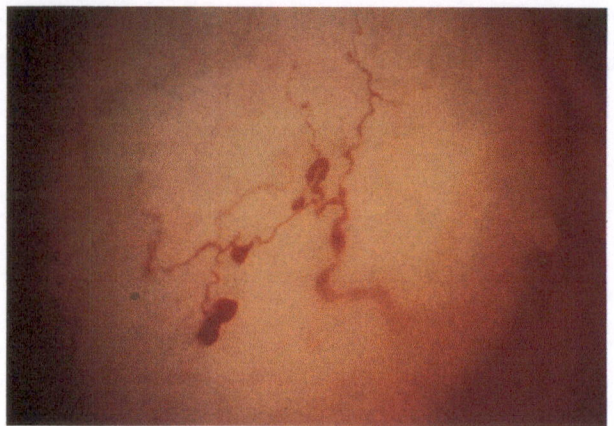

FIGURE 60-1.
Clinical photograph depicts the dilated abnomal conjunctival vessels.

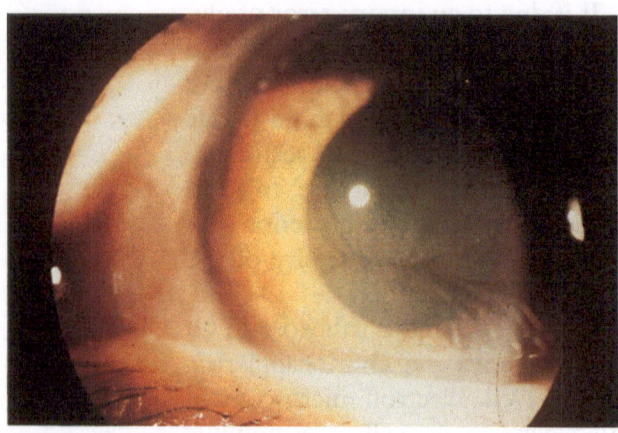

FIGURE 60-2.
Clinical corneal photograph of a patient with Fabry's disease demonstrates the typical cornea verticillata seen with this condition.

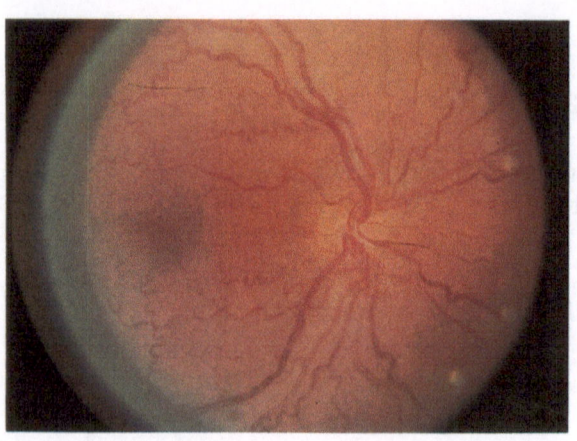

FIGURE 60-3.
Retinal vessels show engorgement and tortuosity.

FIGURE 60-4.

Electron microscopy of a conjunctival biopsy specimen demonstrates the abnormal metabolite in the endothelial cells. (arrows)

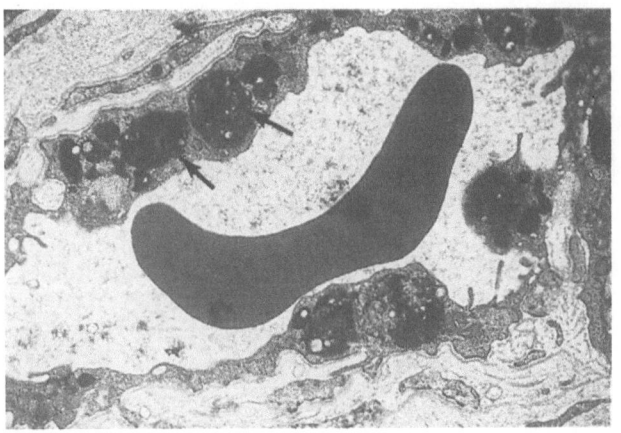

Chapter 61

Tay-Sachs Disease

Tay-Sachs disease, which is inherited in an autosomal recessive manner, is a fatal disease. It is characterized by the absence or deficiency of the enzyme hexosaminidase A. This biochemical defect results in an abnormal deposition of gangliosidase in the central nervous system and the liver. Statistically, it is common in Ashkenazic Jews, and the carrier state for the disease may be 1 in every 30 Jewish people. It has also been reported in children of French-Canadian ancestry. It is possible to assay the levels of the enzyme in amniotic fluid; and, as such, it is commonly tested for when amniocentesis is performed.

At birth the child may appear normal, and the cherry red spot often associated with this disease may be absent. By the time the child is 6 months old, however, neurological signs begin to appear. Classically, the child exhibits hypotonia, optic atrophy, and nystagmus. With time, the ganglion cells are destroyed, and the cherry red spot resolves. There is a progressive paralysis resulting in the death of the infant within the first 24 months of life.

A variant is juvenile Tay-Sachs disease in which the enzyme level is normal or slightly reduced. Such children exhibit visual disturbances, seizures, and progressive deterioration of both mental and motor capacities during the first decade of life. Unlike typical Tay-Sachs disease, where the electroretinogram (ERG) is normal, the juvenile form demonstrates a pronounced change in fundus pigment. As such, one would expect an abnormal ERG and electrooculogram.

Histologically, the ganglion cell cytoplasm is swollen, especially in the macula. The cytoplasm contains periodic acid-Schiff-positive material.

Selected Reading

Cogan DG, Kuwabara T (1959). Histochemistry of the retina in Tay-Sachs disease. Arch Ophthalmol 61:414-423

Ghosh M, Hunter WS, Wedge C (1990). Corneal changes in Tay-Sachs disease. Can J Ophthalmol 25:190-192

Kivlin JD, Sanborn GE, Meyers GG (1985). The cherry-red spot in Tay-Sachs and other storage diseases. Ann Neurol 17:356-360

Figures

FIGURE 61-1.
This child appeared normal at birth. Two other siblings had Tay-Sachs disease, and the parents wanted to know if this child had been spared. Although the child appeared normal during the perinatal period, at 8 months the typical cherry red spot became apparent.

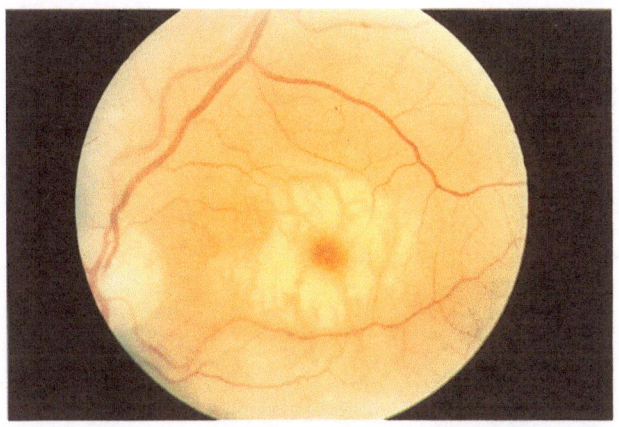

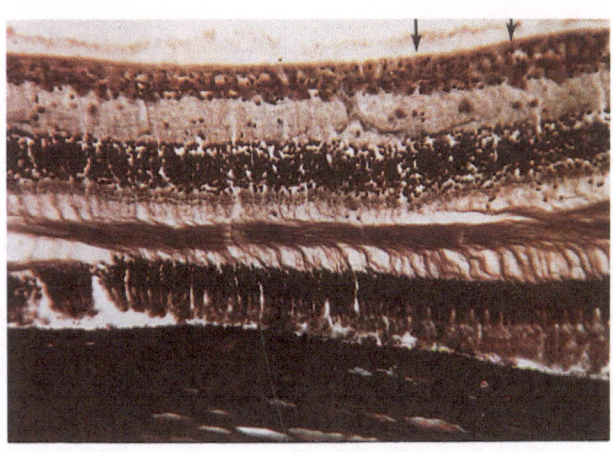

FIGURE 61-2.
In this pathology specimen the ganglion cells are swollen with intracytoplasmic material. (arrows) (H & E)

Index